THERAPEUTIC
YOGA

THERAPEUTIC
YOGA

IN EASY-TO-FOLLOW COLOUR ILLUSTRATIONS BASED
ON THE TEACHINGS OF YOGĀCHĀRYA B.K.S. IYENGAR

Dr. J. T. SHAH

Vakils, Feffer and Simons Ltd.
Hague Building, 9 Sprott Road, Ballard Estate
Mumbai 400 001, India

First printing 1999
Second printing 2001

Price in India

Published by Mrs. Jean Trindade
for Vakils, Feffer and Simons Ltd.
Hague Building, 9 Sprott Road,
Ballard Estate, Mumbai 400 001, India

Printed by Arun K. Mehta at Vakil & Sons (Pvt.) Ltd.
Industry Manor, Appasaheb Marathe Marg,
Worli, Mumbai 400 025.

ISBN No. 81-87111-28-3

My Pranams to

Yogāchārya B. K. S. Iyengar

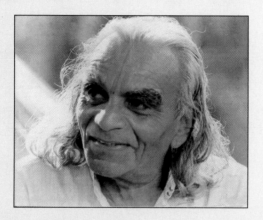

and to

Geetaji and Prasanthji

without whose guidance and blessings

this book would not have been possible

My Homage to
Sage Patañjali

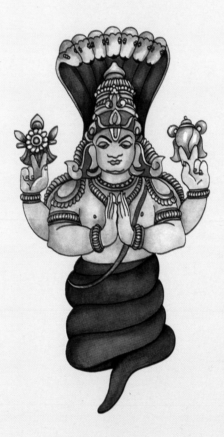

Father of Yoga

Foreword
by
Yogāchārya B. K. S. Iyengar

Today, interest in health consciousness is attracting people from all over the world to earn better health in body and contentment in mind.

The search for health and happiness has opened new avenues in the alternative systems of medicine, as conventional medicine is not helping people to gain physical fitness and mental poise.

Secondly, people are looking towards natural ways of approach in health and happiness. This search has brought <u>YOGA</u> into the limelight and has earned a place in the medical system with its therapeutic value in keeping the inner body and inner mind clean and clear to lead a life of benevolence.

Particularly, the evolutory aspects of yoga, namely āsanas, prāṇāyāmas and dhyāna cultivate moral health, social health, physico-physiological health and psycho-spiritual health.

I am delighted that my pupil Dr. J. T Shah has brought out this book which explains a therapeutic approach of yoga, for maintenance of physical and physiological health as well as poise in mind through these few basic āsanas and prāṇāyāma with minimum techniques and effects. If one further excavates the immeasurable depth of the body with perfection and precision in performing the āsanas and prāṇāyāmas with the subtlest of adjustments, the wisdom of the body is tapped fully to bring health to the surface like the water of a river that runs with ever freshness and power.

Dr. J. T. Shah has also given a new dimension with colour codes as a ready reference for a practitioner to understand the position of the organs, endocrine glands, muscles and joints and then to chose the āsanas for a workout to keep the various systems of the human body in balance, harmony and concord.

I wish the author all success in his attempt in presenting this therapeutic yoga for the good of all.

B. K. S. Iyengar

Acknowledgements

I wish to offer my sincere and profuse thanks to:

- Mr. Arun and Mrs. Sudha Mehta of Vakil and Sons Ltd. for helping me in the publication of this book and for the excellence in printing.

- Dr. Nishit Shah, my son, in helping me with the computer work right from the inception of the book to its completion.

- Dr. Rajeshwar Singh in helping with the editing of the script and for his professional advice.

- Mrs. Sangita Wakode for her help in preparing the artistic drawings of the āsanas.

- Mr. S. Shivagurunathan for his help in preparation of the manuscript.

- Rest of the staff in Vakil and Sons Ltd. for their help in the publication of this book.

- Mrs. Shilpa Shah for her support and professional advice.

- All my family members and friends who encouraged me and helped me to carry out this project.

Dr. J. T. Shah
India House No. 2
Kemp's Corner,
Mumbai 400 036
India.
E-mail : jtshah@bom5.vsnl.net.in

Contents

ĀSANAS
STANDING ĀSANAS

SITTING ĀSANAS

BALANCING ĀSANAS

ĀSANAS IN LYING POSITIONS

Contents

Preface

Today, there is a growing and mature awareness that personal health and happiness are inextricably entwined. Ironically, increasing health consciousness has kept pace with an increase in stress and bodily disorders. The resultant quest for health has more than ever before focused the attention of the west on the Indian System of Yoga.

In its land of birth, yoga is enjoying a newfound respect, this time from a generation looking beyond yoga as 'good exercise'. The young, the healthy, the not- so-young and the not-so-healthy, even the patient and the doctor are acknowledging, that understanding "how yoga works" means understanding how the body and the mind can work better. How to help your body and mind to work better for you through yoga, is what I am setting out to do. This book therefore, is primarily meant to introduce people to the art of yoga and to its therapeutic effects on medical disorders. However, one should not forget that the primary aim of yoga is to achieve self-realization and that the medical benefits are additional effects.

It is recommended that while special emphasis may be put on selected āsanas or yogic postures pertaining to a person's disease, the body must be treated as a whole and an attempt must be made to learn a fuller range of āsanas. However, specific āsanas related to the individual's problems must be done more regularly and the posture held for a longer duration to achieve greater benefit than general āsanas done for the rest of the body. It is also absolutely ɪ ɛcessary to incorporate breath and mind into the āsana to attain maximum benefit.

Prāṇāyāma is breath control. It is intimately linked with oxygenation of blood and therefore has effects which reaches right down to the cellular level thereby improving the functions of all systems.

Meditation is a technique to control the fluctuations of the mind which helps in creating peace and tranquility in the mind. These good effects in turn help to stabilize and balance all other systems.

Yoga, especially āsanas, prāṇāyāma and meditation, can play an important part in both prevention and cure of diseases, as well as in the upliftment of a person's health.

This book gives the main steps of the āsanas to support and supplement the initial training given by the yoga teacher.

Colours have been added to the āsanas or postures to familiarize people with the widespread effects of each āsana on various organs and systems as well as on the mind. Colours will also facilitate the readers to visualize organs and glands involved in a particular āsana, which will enable him/her to custom design a programme of āsanas suited to the problem or disorder of the individual. I am sure that colours will make yoga more colourful and interesting and will widen its popularity in people who are looking towards alternative medicine to cure them. The challenge before us in the health and medical profession is to review our perspective through a new holistic approach and to return to our patients and humanity at large, the equilibrium of mind and body.

Pill popping enthusiasts are urged to restrain their impulse to resort to antibiotics, analgesics and tranquilizers and to adapt instead a sound yoga programme for a long life, with a young body, an alert mind and calm relaxed nerves.

Mumbai   May, 1999   **Dr. J. T. SHAH**

General Instructions

The best time to practice yoga is on an empty stomach, ideally early morning before breakfast. At any other time, it should be done on a fairly empty stomach i.e. two hours after a light meal or four hours after a heavy meal.

Meals can be taken about half an hour after a heavy session or light snacks after about fifteen minutes.

Practice regularly for at least half an hour daily preferably at the same time.

Dress should be loose and comfortable.

Practice with bare feet.

Practice in a warm, quiet, clean and airy place.

Remove glasses and contact lenses before practice.

Empty the bladder before practice.

Avoid practising āsanas during menstrual periods.

Start the session with 5 minutes of toning up exercises to loosen the joints and the body.

Do standing āsanas first, followed by sitting, lying and inverted āsanas, backward bends, twists and forward bends. End the session with 5 minutes of Śavāsana. This is the sequence in which the āsanas have been arranged in this book and therefore after selecting all the āsanas, one has only to start with the āsana selected in the front pages and do the other āsanas following it as you turn the pages. **In every group, easy āsanas must precede the moderately difficult ones, which must precede the difficult ones, keeping a gap of few weeks or months between them. This is the order of arrangement in this book for every group.** However this order of practising āsanas is flexible and can be varied under the guidance of your yoga teacher according to one's needs, experience, physical and mental condition.

In all āsanas in which the right or left side of the body is stretched, bent or twisted more than the other, the opposite side must also be done in a similar way to equally balance the effect.

Āsanas must be done slowly, smoothly and with full understanding.

Practice āsanas with full concentration and awareness of the body parts involved in a given āsana.

Incorporate breathing while going into or coming out of the āsana, as well as while holding of the āsana. Breathe out during all forward bending movements in which the chest or the abdomen is being compressed, and breathe in during all backward bending movements in which the chest or the abdomen is being expanded. The breath and the movement of going

into and coming out of the āsana must be synchronised. Breathe normally while maintaining the pose, with full awareness of the breath.

Maintain the pose as long as you can without any physical or mental strain. The longer the duration of the pose, greater will be the beneficial effect. However the duration of the pose can be decided depending on the time available and on the number of āsanas one wishes to perform.

All forward bending āsanas in which the head is supported are stress relieving āsanas.

Coming out of the pose must be done by retracing the steps of going into the āsana.

Do not force yourself into any final pose. Know your own limitations.

If practising in a group do not compete with others.

If you have any medical problem consult your specialist doctor as well as inform your yoga teacher about the same, before joining the class.

Āsanas and prāṇāyāma may be done after due modification by taking guidance from an experienced yoga teacher in serious cardiovascular, respiratory, orthopedic and other systemic disorders.

Persons with high myopia and those suffering from hypertension, glaucoma, detachment of retina, discharging ears and cervical spondylitis must avoid inverted āsanas. During learning, sarvangasana should be learnt before sirsasana, whilst during practise, sirsasana precedes sarvangasana.

In cervical spondylitis, these may be done by using supports and with the guidance of an experienced teacher.

A warm bath before and 15 minutes after the session will help people who have severe arthritis.

Beneficial effects will be observed after 3 months of regular and sincere practice and even more so after 6 months.

Prāṇāyāma should be done early in the morning atleast one hour prior to an āsana session. Kumbhaka or stoppage of breath must not be done by persons with heart or lung problems or in case of insomnia, poor memory and concentration.

Meditation should be done first thing in the morning, about half an hour before the prāṇāyāma session and / or at night just before retiring.

Abbreviations

Different letters and colours have been selected to represent different systems, organs and tissues in the body, on which the āsana has beneficial effect.

C → Cardiovascular system

E → Endocrine Glands

     AD • adrenals

     G • gonads (ovaries & testes)

     I • islets of Langerhans in pancreas

     PI • pituitary

     PN • pineal

     T • thyroid and parathyroid

     TY • thymus

F → Fat

J → Joints

M → Muscles

N → Nervous system and Mind

O → Organs

A • abdominal organs	K • kidney	P • pelvic organs
C • ear	L • lung	V • voice box or larynx
H • heart		

S → Spine

Using the Book . . .

This book employs colour coding to facilitate customization of the āsanas for any individual or for any given disease condition.

The most prominent effects of the āsana on various tissues, organs or systems are shown by different colour tones in small circles (colour locator) in the right hand corner of the āsana. The extent of beneficial effects of the āsanas has been shown by the size of the circle, the largest circle indicating a maximum effect on that system and small sized circles indicating a relatively lesser effect on other systems. eg.

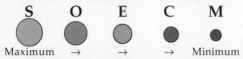

Maximum → → → Minimum

In the above colour locator, the spine (S), organs (O), endocrine glands (E), cardiovascular system (C) and the muscular system (M) are benefitted with the spine receiving the maximum benefit and the muscular system receiving relatively the least benefit.

A letter inside the green circle indicates which organs benefit the most from that āsana. e.g.

 for abdominal organs   for pelvic organs,

 for lungs   for voice box or larynx

Brown and deep blue lines side by side e.g. ▬▬ in the āsana indicate muscular relaxation.

Āsanas have been divided into 3 categories:

     EA -   Easy to perform
     MD -   Moderately Difficult to perform
     DI   -   Difficult to perform

These have been shown in a box in the left hand corner of the āsana and a tick (✔) has been placed in the category to which the āsana belongs. e.g.

EA	MD	DI✔

1. (a) Select āsana from the colour locator kept on the right hand corner of each āsana page depending on which system you would like to strengthen or to help cure any disease condition from which you are suffering.

OR

     (b) Select āsanas from charts (p. xvi, xviii or xix) which give the colour codes as well as page numbers of important āsanas for strengthening a particular system or to help cure any disease conditions or symptoms.

2. After selecting the āsanas, the easier ones in each group must be done for a few weeks or months before proceeding to the moderately difficult ones. A similar gap must be kept before proceeding from the moderately difficult to the difficult āsanas.

3. Follow the advice given in the general instruction (p. xii & xiii).

4. Follow the main steps given on page opposite the āsana and review the benefits and indications given below it.

Āsanas to Benefit Various Systems

	Colour Code	Page Nos. of Important Āsanas & Prāṇāyāmas
Respiratory System	L	12, 32, 34, 44, 46, 60, 66, 70, 74, 96, 98
Cardiovascular System	●	10, 30, 42, 52, 54, 56, 64, 94, 98
Gastro-intestinal System	A	18, 24, 26, 42, 48, 66, 70, 82, 86, 88, 90, 92
Genito-urinary System	P	22, 24, 28, 36, 54, 60, 62, 68, 70, 92
Skeletal System:		
Spine	●	62, 66, 68, 70, 74, 78, 82, 86, 88, 90
Joints	●	16, 22, 32, 34, 38, 40, 50, 76, 82, 84
Endocrine System	●	26, 48, 52, 54, 56, 64, 68, 74, 88, 92
Equilibratory System	e	2, 16, 20, 30, 38, 40, 58
Muscular System .... (to increase stamina)	●	4, 6, 8, 14, 16, 20, 30, 38, 40, 54
Phonatory System (Voice)	V	12, 18, 34, 48, 52, 66, 72, 74, 82
Nervous System and Mind .... (to reduce stress)	●	42, 44, 46, 50, 56, 94, 96, 98, 100

Organs & Endocrine Glands

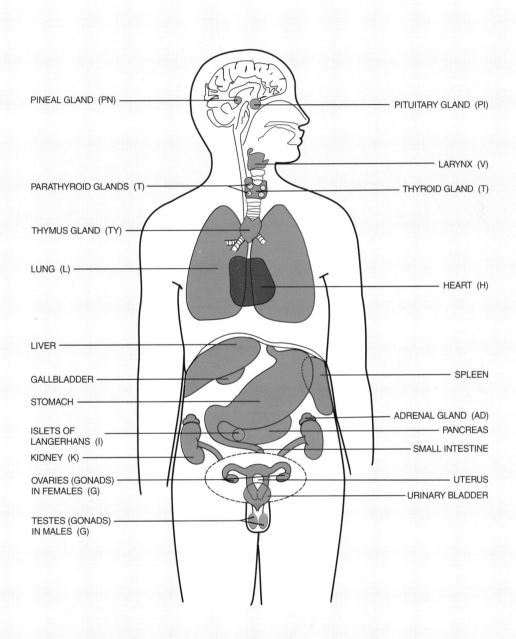

PINEAL GLAND (PN)

PITUITARY GLAND (PI)

LARYNX (V)

PARATHYROID GLANDS (T)

THYROID GLAND (T)

THYMUS GLAND (TY)

LUNG (L)

HEART (H)

LIVER

SPLEEN

GALLBLADDER

STOMACH

ADRENAL GLAND (AD)

PANCREAS

ISLETS OF
LANGERHANS (I)

SMALL INTESTINE

KIDNEY (K)

OVARIES (GONADS)
IN FEMALES (G)

UTERUS

URINARY BLADDER

TESTES (GONADS)
IN MALES (G)

Āsanas that help to cure
disease conditions and symptoms

Diseases and Symptoms	Group of Āsanas, Prāṇāyāmas and Meditation	Colour Code with page no. of important Āsanas and Prāṇāyāmas
Arthritis, Backaches and Spondylitis	Backward bends, Twists, Stress reducing āsanas	16, 42, 44, 50, 66, 68, 70, 74, 76, 78
Asthma, Bronchitis, Bronchiectasis, Chronic lung obstruction, Chronic idiopathic coughs and colds	Backward bends, Forward bends, Stress reducing āsanas, Ujjāyī and Nādī śodhana prāṇāyāma **without retention of breath**	42, 44, 54, 66, 70, 78, 88, 90, 92, 96, 98
Blood pressure – High	Forward bends **with head resting on support,** Stress reducing āsanas, Nādī śodhana prāṇāyāma **without retention of breath** and Meditation	26, 42, 88, 94, 98, 100, 102
Blood pressure – Low	Forward bends, Backward bends, Inverted āsanas, Nādī śodhana prāṇāyāma **without retention of breath**	10, 18, 52, 54, 56, 64, 66, 70, 74, 76, 78
Cerebral Conditions: Insomnia, migraine, poor concentration and memory	Inverted āsanas, Stress reducing āsanas, Ujjāyī and Nādī śodhana prāṇāyāma **without retention of breath** and Meditation	10, 42, 52, 54, 56, 64, 94, 98, 100
Diabetes	Forward bends, Backward bends, Twists, Stress reducing āsanas	26, 44, 48, 62, 66, 82, 88, 90, 98

Diseases and Symptoms	Group of Āsanas, Prāṇāyāmas and Meditation	Colour Code with page no. of important Āsanas and Prāṇāyāmas
Dyspepsia, Constipation Peptic ulcers	Forward bends, Stress reducing āsanas, Nādī śodhana prāṇāyāma	(A) (●) 24, 26, 42, 44, 48, 58, 88, 90, 92, 94, 96, 98
Hyperacidity	Forward bends **with head resting on support** and Stress relieving āsanas	(A) (●) 24, 26, 42, 46, 50, 88, 90, 94, 98, 102
Menstrual disorders: dsymenorrhoea (painful periods), irregular periods	Forward bends, Stress reducing āsanas, Ujjāyī and Nādī śodhana prāṇāyāma. **Avoid āsanas during periods**	(P) (●) 22, 24, 26, 42, 44, 50, 56, 88, 90
Obesity	Standing āsanas, Forward bends, Backward bends, and Twists	(○) 16, 32, 36, 48, 58, 78, 80, 82, 86
Stress related disorders: peptic ulcer, ulcerative colitis, asthma, angina, cardiac arrhymias, diabetes, migraine	Stress reducing āsanas, Nādī śodhana prāṇāyāma **without retention of breath** and Meditation	(●) 42, 44, 46, 50, 88, 94, 98, 100
Voice disorders: vocal hyperfunction and hypofunction disorders	Forward bends, Backward bends, Inverted and Stress removing āsanas. Ujjāyī and Nādī śodhana prāṇāyāma and Meditation	(V) (L) (●) 12, 18, 34, 52, 66, 70, 74, 94, 96, 98, 100

TĀḌĀSANA

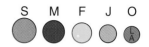

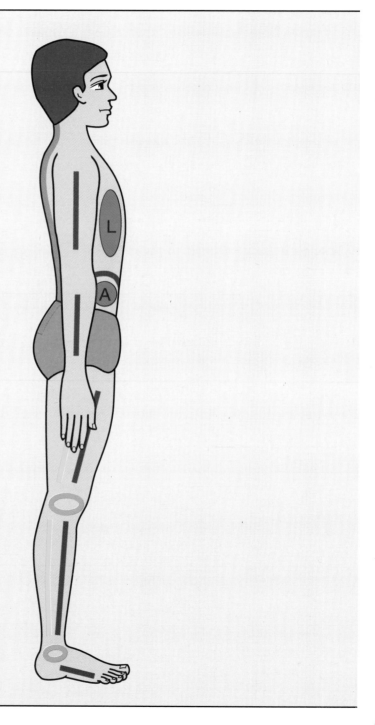

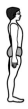

TĀḌĀSANA

ताडासन

Mountain Pose

Main Steps	Stand upright with feet together.
	Keep arms, legs and back straight.
	Keep abdomen tucked in, with chest forward and shoulders braced backwards.
	Maintain the pose and breathe normally.
Benefits	Straightens the spine.
	Strengthens muscles of abdomen and extremities.
	Broadens shoulders and chest.
	Reduces fat around thighs and abdomen.
	Strengthens joints of lower extremities.
	Tones abdominal organs.
Indications	Postural deformities of spine
	Faulty postures and gait
	Weakness of legs
	Obesity of thighs and abdomen
	Drooping shoulders
	Visceroptosis (sagging abdominal organs)
	Narrow chest

VṚKṢĀSANA

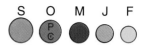

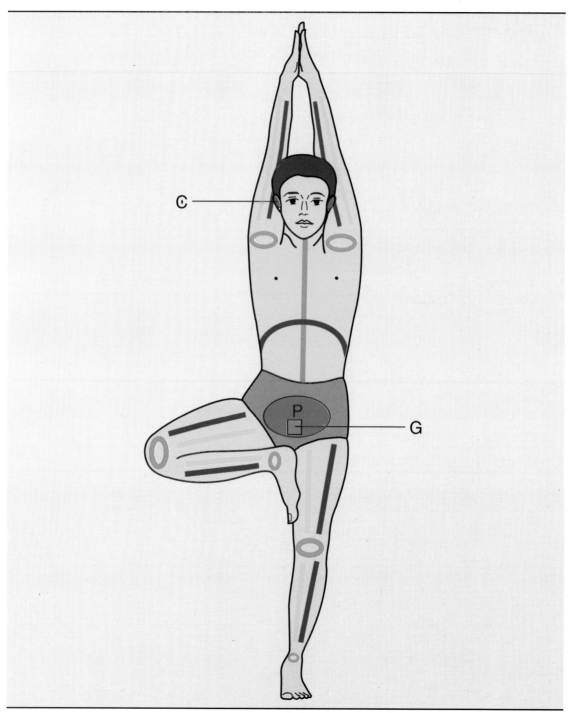

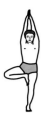

VṚKṢĀSANA

वृक्षासन

Tree Pose

Main Steps	Stand in Tāḍāsana (p. 1).
	Take right leg up and place foot on left thigh as high as possible, toes pointing down.
	Keep left leg absolutely straight, with knee locked.
	Balance and keep hands in prayer position.
	Inhale and raise both hands up straight over the head, palms facing each other.
	Maintain the pose and breathe normally.
	Exhale and return to original pose.
Benefits	Straightens the spine.
	Strengthens inner ears and eyes.
	Improves balance.
	Improves tone in leg muscles.
	Strengthens the knee and loosens the hip joints.
	Strengthens the shoulders.
Indications	Postural deformities of spine
	Mild giddiness
	Weakness of legs and shoulders
	Arthritis of joints of upper and lower extremities

UTKAṬĀSANA

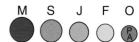

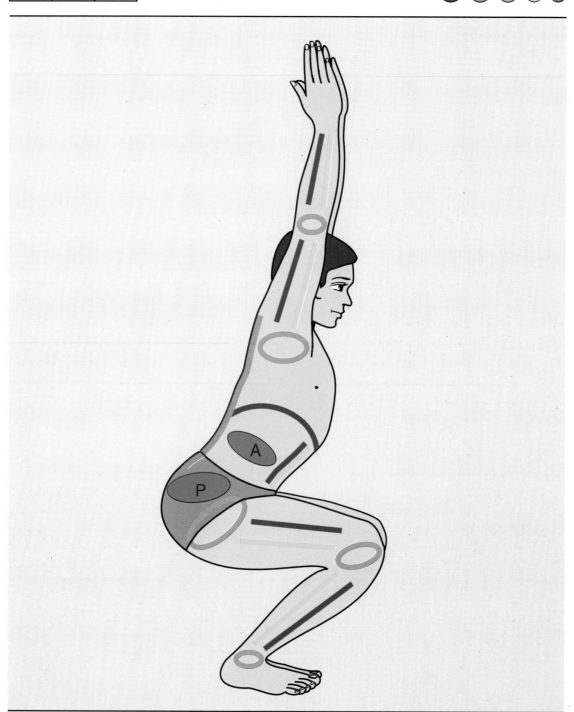

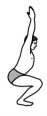

UTKAṬĀSANA

उत्कटासन

Powerful Pose

Main Steps	Stand in Tāḍāsana (p. 1).
	Inhale and stretch arms straight up, palms facing each other.
	Exhale, bend knees and lower the trunk so that thighs are parallel to the floor.
	Keep back straight, chest as far back as possible, and feet flat on ground.
	Maintain posture and breathe normally.
	Inhale and resume erect posture.
	Exhale and bring arms down to normal position.
Benefits	Strengthens muscles of upper and lower extremities, abdomen and diaphragm.
	Strengthens feet and toes.
	Tones the spine.
	Strengthens ankle, knee, hip and shoulder joints.
	Reduces fat in thighs and calves.
	Massages pelvic organs.
	Improves stamina.
Indications	Weakness of legs and abdominal muscles
	Weakness of spine
	Arthritis of upper and lower extremity
	Obesity
	Genito-urinary disorders of urinary bladder, uterus, ovaries, testes and prostate

VĪRABHADRĀSANA - II

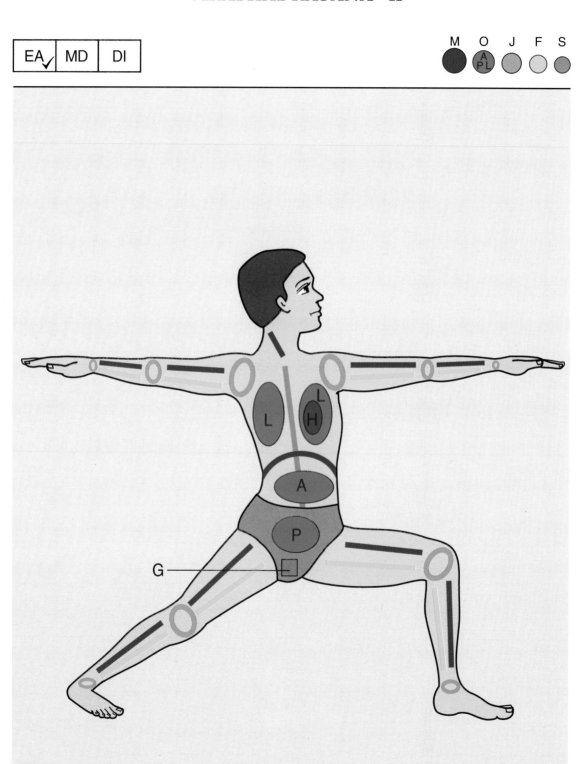

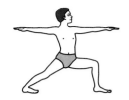

VĪRABHADRĀSANA-II

वीरभद्रासन

Virbhadra's Pose II

Main Steps	Stand in Tāḍāsana (p. 1).
	Inhale and jump 4 feet apart and keep arms parallel to floor.
	Turn left foot out 90° and right foot in 30°.
	Bend left leg to a right angle, allowing the torso to descend vertically downwards at the same spot with navel pointing forwards.
	Look towards the left and gaze at the fingers of the left hand.
	Maintain the pose and breathe normally.
	Inhale and return to the original position by retracing the steps in the reverse order.
	Repeat pose on opposite side.
Benefits	Strengthens leg, thigh, abdominal and neck muscles.
	Tones abdominal and pelvic organs.
	Removes stiffness from all joints.
	Reduces fat around arms and thighs.
	Elongates and strengthens the spine.
	Improves stamina.
Indications	Weakness of arms and legs
	Disorders of abdominal and pelvic organs
	Arthritis
	Obesity involving arms, thighs or abdomen
	Stiffness of spine

UTTHITA TRIKOṆĀSANA

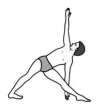

UTTHITA TRIKONĀSANA

उत्थित त्रिकोणासन

Extended Triangle Pose

Main Steps	Stand in Tāḍāsana (p. 1).
	Inhale and jump 3 feet apart.
	Raise arms to a horizontal level and keep them parallel to the floor.
	Turn left foot out 90° and right foot in 30°.
	Exhale and bend trunk towards the left and allow left palm to rest on the floor, close to and behind the left heel.
	Raise right arm up in line with the opposite shoulder.
	Look towards the right thumb.
	Maintain the pose and breathe normally.
	Inhale and return to original pose retracing the steps in a reverse order.
	Repeat the pose on the opposite side.
Benefits	Tones abdominal and respiratory organs.
	Strengthens spine and the neck.
	Tones muscles of the side of chest, abdomen and legs.
	Strengthens ankle, knee and shoulder joints.
	Reduces fat around waist and thighs.
	Improves stamina and balance.
Indications	Gastro-intestinal disorders of stomach, liver, spleen and intestines
	Respiratory disorders: chronic bronchitis and asthma
	Backaches and spondylitis
	Weakness of legs
	Weak ankles and knee joints
	Broad waist and thighs

UTTĀNĀSANA

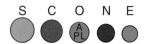

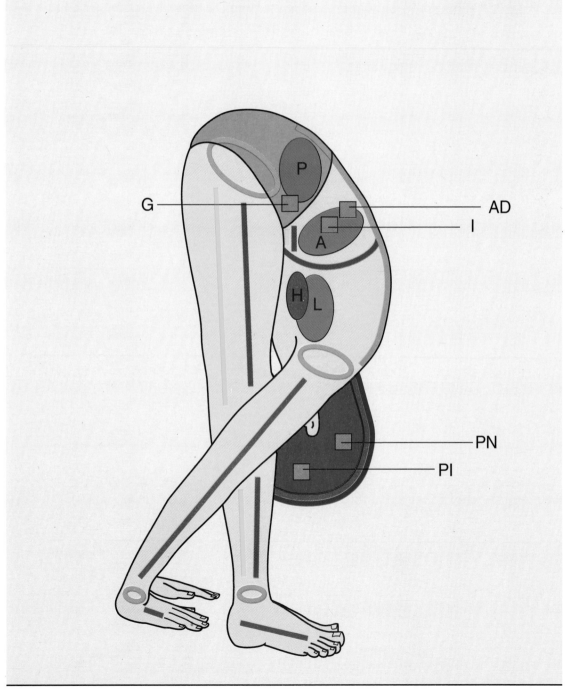

UTTĀNĀSANA

उत्तानासन

Spine Stretching Pose

Main Steps	Stand in Tāḍāsana (p. 1).
	Inhale, extend arms up along the sides and face palms forwards.
	Exhale, bend trunk and extended arms forwards and downwards and allow hands to touch floor or place palms on floor.
	Exhale and allow trunk to move closer to legs and the head to sink downwards and rest forehead on the shins.
	Keep both legs erect and perpendicular to floor and nape of neck totally relaxed.
	Maintain the pose and breathe normally.
	Inhale and return to original pose.
Benefits	Stretches spine.
	Improves blood flow to head and neck.
	Improves blood flow to hypothalamus, pituitary, pineal, thyroid, parathyroid and thymus glands.
	Massages abdominal and pelvic organs.
	Soothes nerves and calms the mind.
	Tones gonads.
	Loosens hip and shoulder joints.
	Strengthens and slims thighs and calves.
Indications	Stiffness of spine
	Physical and mental fatigue or exhaustion
	Giddiness and low blood pressure
	Gastro-intestinal disorders of stomach, intestines, liver, gall bladder, spleen and pancreas
	Genito-urinary disorders of urinary bladder, uterus and prostate
	Pituitary, thyroid and parathyroid disorders
	Mental depression, insomnia and lack of concentration
	Stiffness of hip and shoulder joints
	Preparatory posture for inverted āsanas

VĪRABHADRĀSANA - I

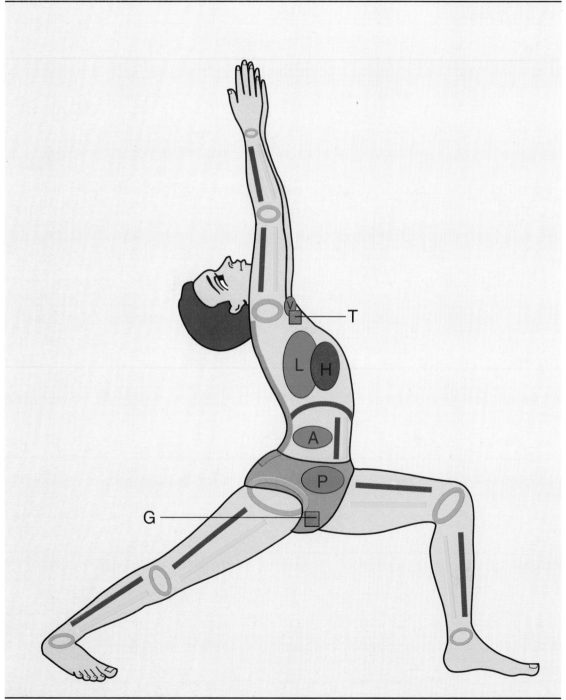

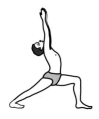

VĪRABHADRĀSANA-I

वीरभद्रासन

Virbhadra's Pose I

Main Steps	Stand in Tāḍāsana (p. 1).
	Inhale and jump 4 feet apart raising both arms to a horizontal level.
	Inhale and raise both arms vertically, palms facing each other.
	Exhale and twist to the left with left foot turning 90° and right foot 30° so that trunk and navel face towards the left.
	Exhale and bend left knee to a right angle and extend head and neck upwards to look towards the ceiling.
	Keep right leg completely stretched and outer border of foot and heel in contact with the floor.
	Maintain the pose and breathe normally.
	Exhale and return to original position by retracing the steps in the reverse order.
	Repeat pose on opposite side.
Benefits	Tones the spine.
	Tones larynx, chest, abdominal and pelvic organs.
	Strengthens leg muscles and improves stamina.
	Strengthens all joints.
	Reduces fat around waist.
	Stimulates thyroid gland.
Indications	Cervical spondylitis
	Voice disorders
	Asthma and bronchitis
	Digestive and pelvic organ disorders
	Menstrual disorders
	Weakness of legs
	Arthritis
	Drooping shoulders
	Obesity of waist, hips and thighs
	Thyroid disorders

UTTHITA PĀRŚVAKOṆĀSANA

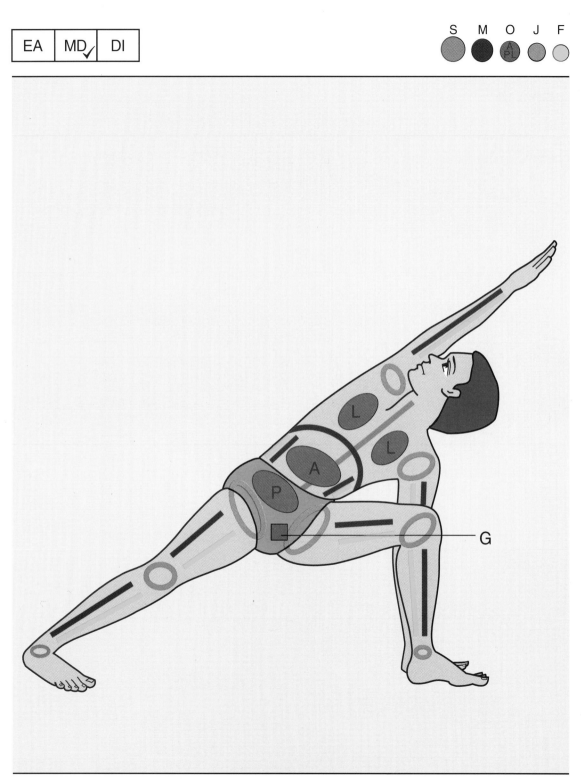

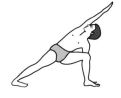

UTTHITA PĀRŚVAKOṆĀSANA

उत्थित पार्श्वकोणासन

Extended Lateral Angle Pose

Main Steps	Stand in Tāḍāsana (p. 1).
	Inhale and jump 4 feet apart, and spread both arms horizontally, parallel to floor.
	Turn left foot out 90° and right foot in 30°.
	Bend left knee to a right angle, allowing trunk to descend vertically.
	Place left hand on the ground close to outer border of left heel and left armpit touching the knee.
	Stretch right hand over the head with palm facing down.
	Look upwards and fix your gaze on a spot on the ceiling.
	Maintain the pose and breathe normally.
	Inhale and return to original position by retracing the steps in the reverse order.
	Repeat pose on opposite side.
Benefits	Stretches and strengthens the spine.
	Strengthens muscles of sides of chest and waist along with those of upper and lower extremities.
	Tones muscles of neck.
	Tones heart, abdominal organs and gonads.
	Strengthens all joints of upper and lower extremities.
	Reduces obesity around waist, arms and legs.
	Increases stamina.
Indications	Spondylitis
	Weakness of upper and lower extremities
	Arthritis
	Obesity of abdomen, arms or hips
	Gastro-intestinal, respiratory and sexual disorders
	General weakness

GARUḌĀSANA

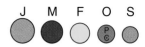

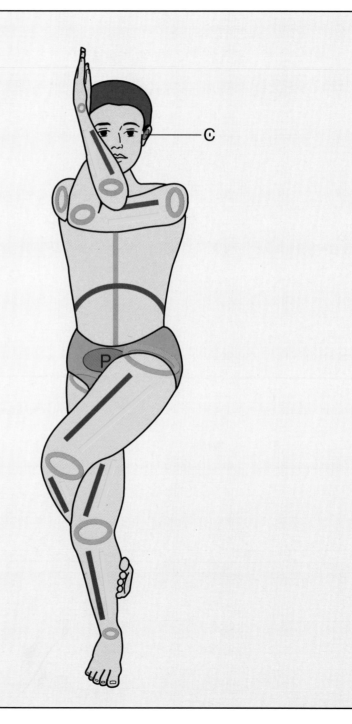

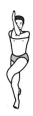

GARUḌĀSANA

गरुडासन

Eagle Pose

Main Steps	Stand in Tāḍāsana (p. 1).
	Bend right knee slightly, and place left thigh over the right.
	Twist left calf around the right, so that left big toe hooks around the inner side of the right calf.
	Cross right elbow over the left, twist left forearm around the right, so that palms come in proximity and face each other.
	Raise arms to shoulder level and straighten and elongate the back.
	Straighten right knee as much as possible.
	Maintain the pose and breathe normally.
	Exhale and return to original pose.
	Repeat pose with the opposite leg and arm in the front.
Benefits	Loosens joints of both extremities.
	Tones and strengthens upper and lower extremities.
	Reduces obesity of arms, calves and thighs.
	Improves balance.
	Stretches the spine.
Indications	Stiffness of joints of upper and lower extremities
	Weakness of legs and arms
	Obesity of arms, thighs and calves
	Mild giddiness
	Stiffness of spine

PĀRŚVOTTĀNĀSANA

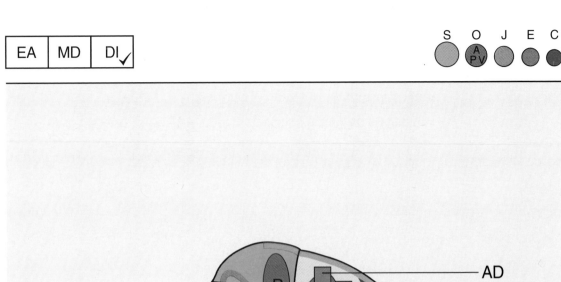

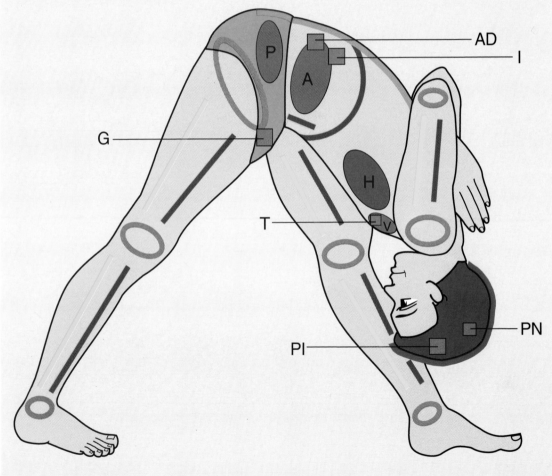

PĀRŚVOTTĀNĀSANA

पाश्वोत्तानासन

Side Stretching Pose

Main Steps	Stand in Tāḍāsana (p. 1).
	Take palms behind the back and join them in prayer position with fingers pointing upwards.
	Take them up as high as possible between the shoulder blades.
	Inhale and jump 4 feet apart.
	Exhale and twist to the left by turning left foot out 90° and right foot in 70°.
	Exhale and bend forward and downward towards the left knee to allow forehead to touch the knee.
	Keep elbows as high as possible to allow palms to remain together and the spine to descend further.
	Maintain the pose and breathe normally.
	Inhale and return to original position by retracing the steps in the reverse order.
	Repeat pose on the opposite side.
Benefits	Tones spine.
	Massages abdominal organs.
	Tones neck and larynx.
	Strengthens all the joints.
	Improves blood flow to brain, head, neck and endocrine glands in brain and neck.
	Reduces fat around thighs and abdomen.
Indications	Stiffness of spine
	Gastro-intestinal disorders of liver, spleen and intestines
	Voice disorders
	Stiffness of joints
	Diabetes and thyroid disorders
	Mental and physical fatigue
	Obesity of thighs and abdomen
	Migraine and insomnia

VĪRABHADRĀSANA - III

S M J O F

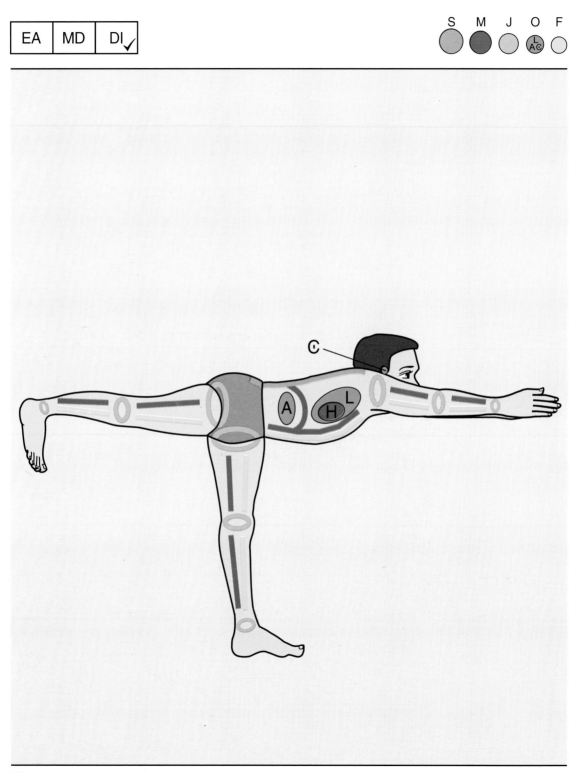

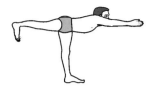

VĪRABHADRĀSANA-III

वीरभद्रासन

Virbhadra's Pose III

Main Steps	Stand in Tāḍāsana (p. 1).

Main Steps

Stand in Tāḍāsana (p. 1).

Inhale and jump 4 feet apart and raise arms and bring palms together.

Exhale and twist to the left, turning left foot out 90° and right foot in 70°.

Exhale and bend left knee to a right angle to be in Vīrabhadrāsana-I (p. 13).

Exhale and bend extended arms and chest forwards, to bring chest in contact with left thigh.

Exhale and lift right leg and straighten left leg simultaneously, so that the trunk, extended arms and right leg are parallel to floor.

Balance body on erect straight left leg, head extended, and eyes looking forward.

Maintain the pose and breathe normally.

Exhale and return to original pose by retracing steps in a reverse order.

Repeat the pose balancing on the opposite leg.

Benefits

Strengthens spine.

Strengthens legs and reduces obesity around thighs, calves and arms.

Strengthens neck, abdominal and back muscles.

Loosens shoulder and hip joints.

Tones abdominal organs.

Improves balance, poise and concentration.

Strengthens inner ears and eyes.

Indications

Spondylitis and backaches

Weak legs

Weak abdominal and back muscles

Arthritis of joints of upper and lower extremities

Gastro-intestinal disorders

Mild giddiness

Obesity of thighs, calves and arms

Weak eyes and ears

BADDHA KOṆĀSANA

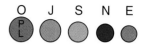

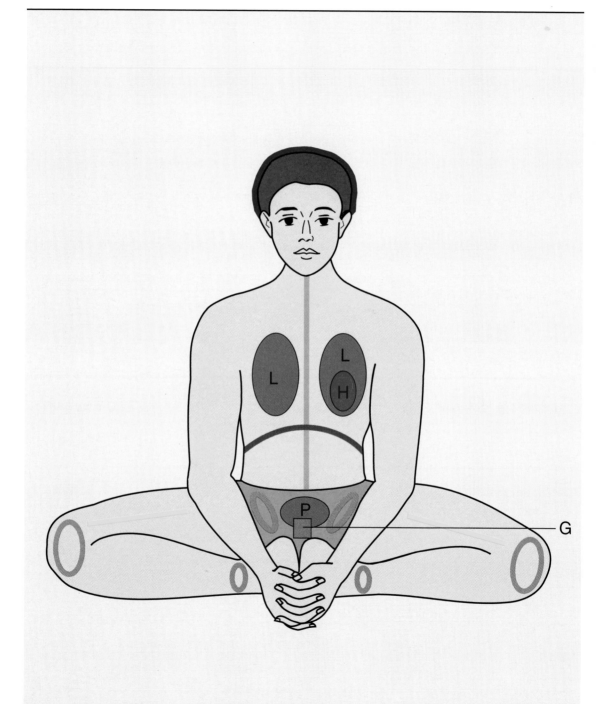

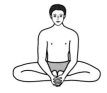

BADDHA KOṆĀSANA

बद्ध कोणासन

Cobbler's Pose

Main Steps	Sit with back erect and legs straight.
	Exhale, bend knees and bring heels as close as possible to genitals.
	Exhale, allow knees to fall on the sides and bring soles and heels of feet in contact with each other.
	Catch feet with hands and allow knees and thighs to go down towards floor by pressing thighs down, with elbows and forearms.
	Straighten the back and look straight ahead with eyes relaxed.
	Maintain the pose and breathe normally.
	Exhale and return to original position.
Benefits	Relieves pelvic congestion and tones pelvic organs.
	Loosens knee and hip joints.
	Straightens the spine.
	Soothes nerves and the mind.
	Tones gonads.
Indications	Genito-urinary disorders of prostate, ovaries, testes and urinary bladder
	Menstrual irregularities
	Arthritis of knee and hip joints
	Sciatica and backaches
	Disorders of sex glands
	Preparatory posture for Padmāsana (p. 29)

VĪRĀSANA

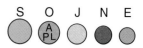

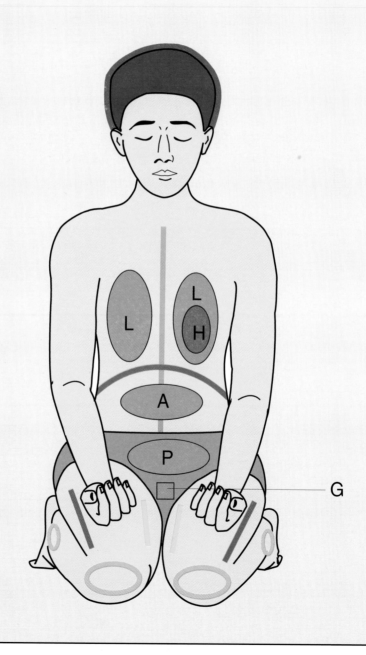

VĪRĀSANA

वीरासन

Hero's Pose

Main Steps	Kneel on the floor with back erect.
	Allow hips to go down and rest them between the feet with toes pointing backwards.
	Keep the back erect and hands resting on the knees palms facing upwards.
	Join index finger with the thumb to form a ring (gyana mudra).
	Maintain the pose and breathe normally.
	Bend forward and rest in Adho Mukha Vīrāsana pose (p. 27)
Benefits	Strengthens spine.
	Tones stomach and improves digestion.
	Massages pelvic organs.
	Improves flexibility of the toes, ankles and the knees.
	Deepens arches of feet.
	Quietens the mind.
	Tones gonads.
	Reduces fat around thighs and calves.
Indications	Weak spine
	Digestive disorders: dyspepsia and indigestion
	Genito-urinary disorders of prostate, uterus, testes and ovaries
	Stiffness of toes, ankles and knees
	Flat feet
	Anxiety and tension states
	Menstrual disorders: dysmenorrhoea (painful periods)
	Fat around thighs and calves

ADHO MUKHA VĪRĀSANA

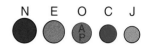

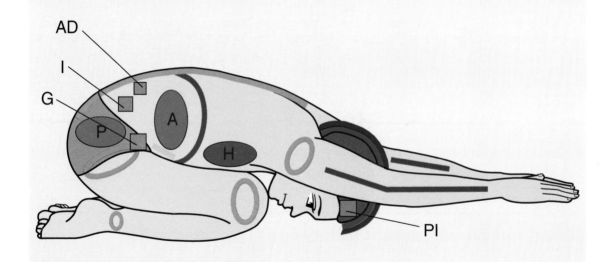

ADHO MUKHA VĪRĀSANA

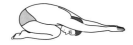

अधो मुख वीरासन

Face Down Hero's Pose

Main Steps	Sit in Vīrāsana (p. 25).
	Spread the knees a little apart and bend trunk and chest forward between them allowing forehead to rest on the floor.
	Extend arms forward to rest on the floor.
	Maintain the pose and breathe normally.
	Inhale and return to original pose.
Benefits	Quietens the mind.
	Removes physical and mental fatigue.
	Tones adrenals and islets of Langerhans.
	Tones abdominal organs.
	Improves blood supply to brain, head and neck.
	Loosens ankle, knee, hip and shoulder joints.
	Reduces stiffness of spine.
Indications	Stress related disorders: asthma, diabetes and hypertension
	General physical or mental fatigue
	Endocrine disorders of islets of Langerhans, adrenals and gonads
	Gastro-intestinal disorders of stomach, intestines, liver, spleen and pancreas
	Genito-urinary disorders of urinary bladder, kidneys, uterus, ovaries and testes
	Menstrual disorders
	Stiffness of knees, hips and ankles
	Stiffness of spine

PADMĀSANA

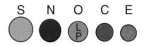

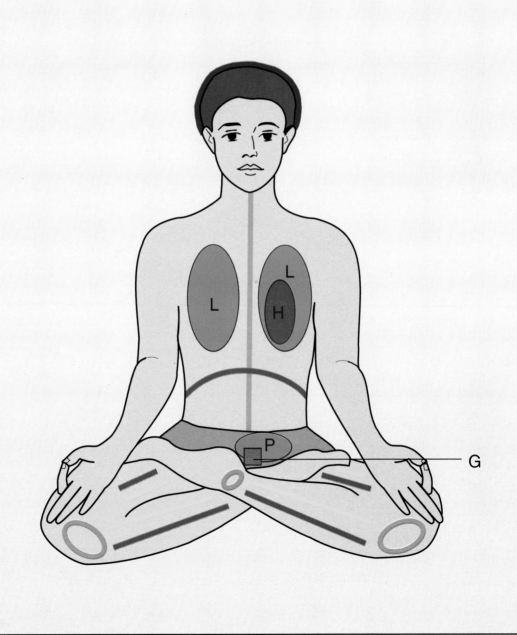

PADMĀSANA

पद्मासन

Lotus Pose

Main Steps	Sit with both feet straight.
	Bend right knee and place outer border of right foot on the left groin.
	Bend left knee and place outer border of left foot on the right groin.
	Try and lift heels further up on the groin and move both knees as close to each other as possible.
	Keep the back straight and shoulders back.
	Rest the hands on the thighs, with the palms facing up, and the index fingers and thumbs forming a ring (gyana mudra).
	Maintain the pose and breathe normally.
	Return to original position by retracing the steps.
Benefits	Tones abdominal organs and spine.
	Tranquillises mind and heart.
	Opens chest and lungs.
	Increases blood flow to pelvic organs and gonads.
	Loosens knees, ankles and hips.
	Reduces fat around thighs and calves.
Indications	Mental stress and strain
	Spondylitis of thoracic and lumbar spine
	Low backaches
	Genito-urinary and prostate disorders
	Stiffness of knees, ankles and hips
	Obesity around thighs and calves

PARIPŪRṆA NĀVĀSANA

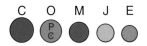

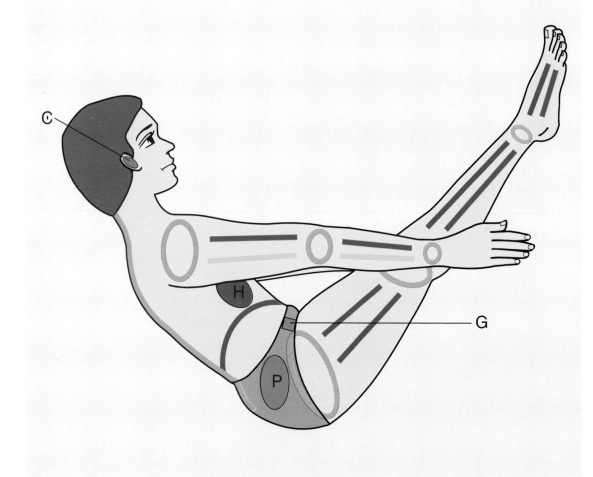

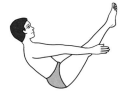

PARIPŪRṆA NĀVĀSANA

परिपूर्ण नावासन

Full Boat Pose

Main Steps	Sit on floor with back erect and legs stretched out in front, with palms on floor, fingers pointing forwards.
	Exhale, lean back and raise legs to 60° from the floor.
	Raise arms straight to shoulder level and parallel to the floor.
	Balance on hips with eyes looking straight ahead.
	Maintain the pose and breathe normally.
	Exhale and lower the legs and the body to a lying position and breathe normally.
Benefits	Reduces load on heart.
	Massages and improves blood flow to abdominal and pelvic organs.
	Increases blood flow to adrenals, islets of Langerhans and gonads.
	Reduces swelling of feet.
	Strengthens thighs and arms.
	Improves balance.
Indications	Angina and early cardiac problems (done with support to legs and back)
	Gastro-intestinal and pelvic organ disorders: diarrhoea, dysentery, colitis, dyspepsia, liver, spleen and pancreatic disorders
	Asthma, diabetes and sexual disorders
	Oedema of feet due to any cause
	Weakness of legs and arms
	Mild giddiness

GOMUKHĀSANA

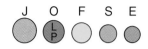

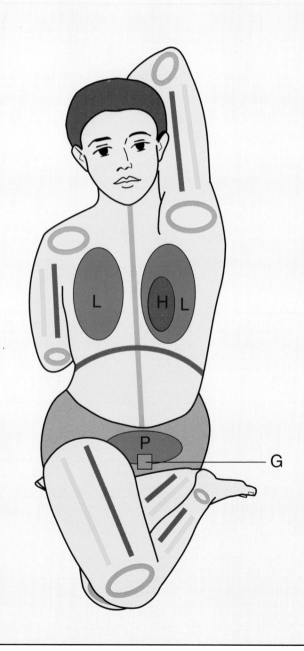

GOMUKHĀSANA

गोमुखासन

Cow's Face Pose

Main Steps	Sit with legs stretched in front and arms on side of hips.
	Raise hips; bend left knee to the left along the floor and place left foot horizontally under the hips.
	Gently sit over it.
	Bend right knee and place right thigh on top of left thigh with outer border of right foot resting horizontally on the floor, toes pointing backwards.
	Keep back erect.
	Raise left arm, bend it at the elbow and place palm facing forward between two shoulder blades.
	Take right arm behind, bend it at the elbow and place palm facing backward between the shoulder blades.
	Grip fingers of both hands and bring hands closer to each other by allowing both elbows to move backwards.
	Maintain the pose and breathe normally.
	Exhale and return to original pose by retracing steps in the reverse order.
	Repeat pose with opposite thigh on top.
Benefits	Loosens all small and big joints.
	Expands chest and lungs.
	Massages and improves blood flow to pelvic organs.
	Reduces obesity in thighs, legs and arms.
	Stretches spine.
	Tones gonads.
	Strengthens shoulders, arms and thighs.
Indications	Arthritis
	Respiratory disorders: asthma, bronchitis and emphysema
	Genito-urinary disorders of urinary bladder, uterus and prostate
	Obesity around thighs, calves and arms
	Stiffness of spine
	Disorders of sex glands
	Weak shoulders, arms and thighs

SIMHĀSANA-II

O   J   E   S   M

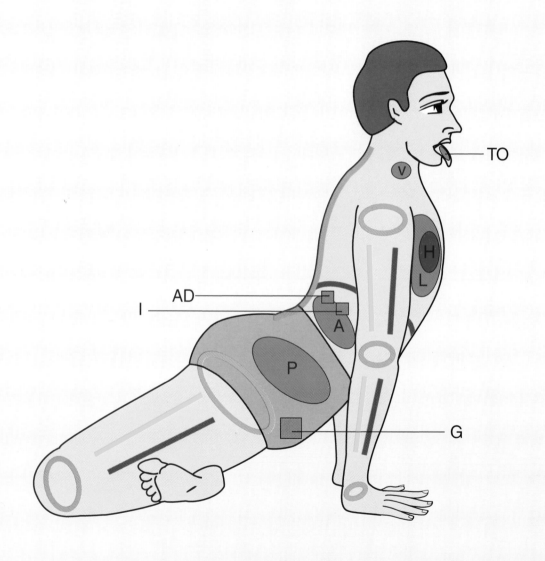

SIMHĀSANA-II

सिंहासन

Lion Pose

Main Steps	Sit in Padmāsana (p. 29).
	Place extended arms on side of thighs and raise trunk up on knees shifting the arms to the front and placing palms on the floor.
	Push pubis forward towards the floor by shifting the palms further forward on the floor to stretch the back and make it concave.
	Open the mouth and stretch the tongue out towards the chin as much as possible.
	Look towards the tip of the nose and breath through the mouth.
	Maintain the pose and breathe.
	Exhale and return to original pose.
	Repeat the pose again with the opposite leg on top in Padmāsana. (p. 29)
Benefits	Tones and clears the tongue, throat and larynx.
	Removes bad breath (halitosis).
	Improves speech.
	Expands chest and lungs.
	Tones abdominal and pelvic organs.
	Strengthens all joints.
	Tones adrenals, islets of Langerhans and gonads.
	Strengthens back muscles and spine.
	Reduces fat around the hips, thighs and arms.
Indications	Tonsillitis, sore throats, laryngitis, halitosis (bad breath)
	Speech and voice disorders
	Respiratory disorders: asthma and bronchitis
	Gastro-intestinal disorders of liver, stomach and intestines
	Genito-urinary disorders of urinary bladder, uterus and prostate
	Arthritis
	Disorders of sexual glands and diabetes
	Stiffness of spine and backaches
	Weak wrists and ankles
	Obesity of thighs, arms and hips

PARĪGHĀSANA

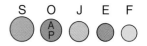

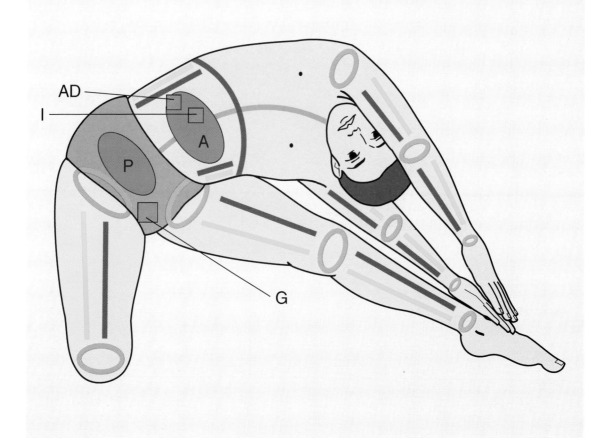

PARĪGHĀSANA

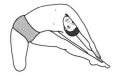

परीघासन

Gate Pose

Main Steps	Kneel on knees with thighs and trunk erect.
	Stretch left leg to left in line with the trunk, knee pointing upwards, and raise both arms up parallel to the floor.
	Exhale, bend trunk and left arm to the left in line with the left leg, and rest the forearm on the shin with palm facing upwards.
	Take right arm over the head with palm facing downwards and touch left palm without bending forward.
	Maintain the pose and breathe normally.
	Repeat pose on the opposite side.
Benefits	Tones up paravertebral muscles and spine.
	Massages abdominal and pelvic organs.
	Strengthens all muscles and joints of upper and lower extremities.
	Tones adrenals, islets of Langerhan and gonads.
	Extends and expands sides of chest and lungs.
	Reduces fat around the waist, thighs and calves.
Indications	Low and mid backaches
	Gastro-intestinal disorders of stomach, liver, spleen and intestines
	Genito-urinary disorders of kidneys, urinary bladder, uterus and prostate
	Arthritis
	Diabetes, asthma and sexual disorders
	Obesity around the waist, thighs and calves
	Weakness of legs

BHUJAPĪḌĀSANA

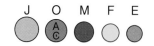

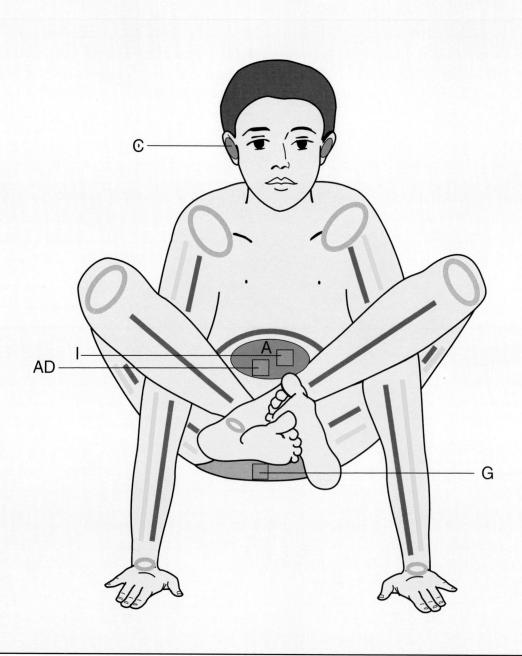

BHUJAPĪḌĀSANA

भुजपीडासन

Knee Shoulder Pose

Main Steps	Stand in Tāḍāsana (p. 1) with feet one foot apart.
	Note: Keep a blanket just behind the feet to avoid hurting the hips, in case balance is lost.
	Bend trunk forward, bend knees and place hands on floor between legs as far back as possible.
	Bring palms forward on outer sides of feet, and rest thighs on upper arm, as high as possible.
	Exhale and raise feet off the floor one at a time, and cross them over each other at the ankles.
	Straighten arms and balance.
	Maintain the pose and breathe normally.
	Exhale and return to original pose by retracing the steps in a reverse order.
	Repeat āsana with opposite foot on top.
Benefits	Strengthens muscles and joints of upper and lower extremities.
	Improves balance, concentration and will power.
	Strengthens inner ears and eyes.
	Tones and strengthens abdominal organs and muscles.
	Tones adrenal glands.
	Reduces obesity of arms and thighs.
Indications	Weakness of upper and lower extremities
	Stiffness of extremity joints
	Lack of concentration and diffidence
	Weak abdominal muscles
	Gastro-intestinal disorders of stomach, intestines, liver and spleen.
	Diabetes
	Obesity of arms and thighs

BAKĀSANA

EA	MD	DI ✓

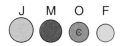

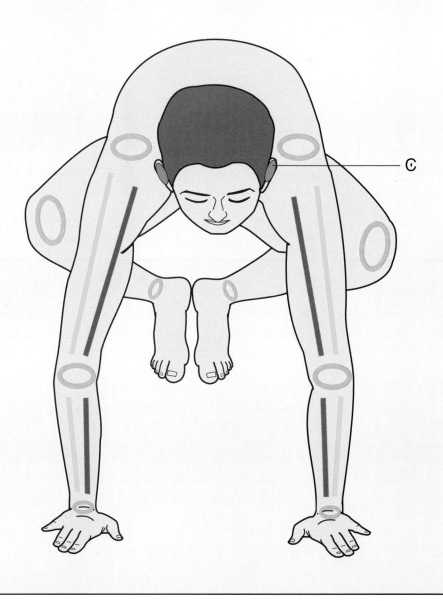

BAKĀSANA

बकासन

Crane Pose

Main Steps	Stand in Tāḍāsana (p. 1).

Main Steps

Stand in Tāḍāsana (p. 1).

Bend the knees and squat.

Note: Keep a blanket in front of the feet to avoid hurting the head, in case balance is lost.

Widen knees, bend trunk forward and allow shins to contact the upper arms.

Widen elbows and place palms on the floor, fingers pointing forward.

Bend trunk and chest further forwards between the arms, raise the hips and heels up, and rest the shins on the arms as high and close to the armpits as possible.

Exhale and lift feet up, one at a time, straighten the arms and balance on hands.

Maintain the pose and breathe normally.

Exhale and return to original position.

Benefits

Improves balance and concentration.

Strengthens muscles and joints of upper extremities, including palms and fingers.

Tones abdominal muscles.

Strengthens inner ears and eyes.

Indications

Stiffness of upper extremity joints

Weak upper extremities

Poor concentration and diffidence

Flabby and weak abdomen

SUPTA BADDHA KOṆĀSANA

EA ✓ | MD | DI

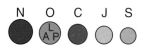

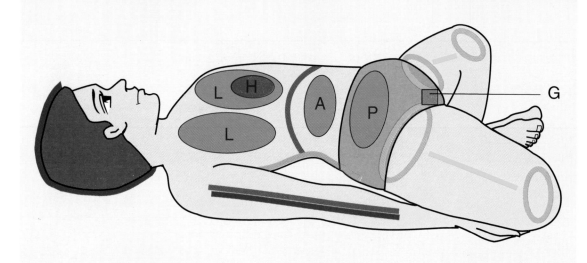

SUPTA BADDHA KOṆĀSANA

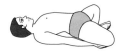

सुप्त बद्ध कोणासन

Cobbler's Pose in Lying Position

Main Steps	Sit in Baddha Koṇāsana (p. 23).
	Recline back and allow head and back to come in contact with floor.
	Push hands under the thighs, hold ankles and pull them up so that the heels touch the anal region.
	Keep outer sides of knees in full contact with the floor.
	Keep arms on side of thighs with palms facing the ceiling.
	Maintain the pose and breathe normally.
	Exhale and return to original pose.
Benefits	Tranquillizes mind.
	Expands chest and lungs.
	Tones abdominal organs.
	Relieves pelvic congestion.
	Relieves congestion in gonads.
	Lowers blood pressure.
	Loosens knee and hip joints.
Indications	General physical or mental fatigue
	Insomnia, anxiety and tension states
	Respiratory disorders: asthma and bronchitis
	Gastro-intestinal disorders: colitis, diarrhoea, dysentery, and peptic ulcer
	Genito-urinary disorders of urinary bladder, uterus, ovaries, testes and prostate
	Menstrual disorders
	Disorders of sex glands
	High blood pressure
	Stiff knee and hip joints

SUPTA VIRĀSANA

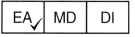

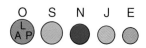

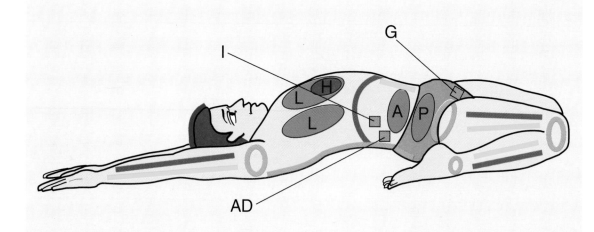

SUPTA VĪRĀSANA

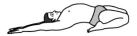

सुप्त वीरासन

Hero's Pose in Lying Position

Main Steps	Sit in Vīrāsana (p. 25).
	Recline back and rest elbows on the floor.
	Extend the arms one at a time and allow the head and the back to rest on the floor.
	Take arms over the head and straighten them.
	Maintain the pose and breathe normally.
	Exhale and return to original pose, lean forwards and rest in Adho Mukha Vīrāsana pose (p. 27).
Benefits	Expands chest and lungs.
	Tones heart and abdominal organs.
	Reduces congestion in pelvic organs.
	Straightens and tones the spine.
	Quietens the mind.
	Loosens ankle, knee, hip and shoulder joints.
	Tones adrenals, islets of Langerhans and gonads.
	Reduces fat around thighs and calves.
Indications	Respiratory disorders: asthma, bronchitis, and chronic obstructive lung disease
	Gastro-intestinal disorders: dyspepsia, diarrhoea and colitis
	Menstrual disorders
	Postural defects of spine
	Anxiety and mental tension
	Stiffness of ankle, knee, hip and shoulder joints
	Endocrine disorders: diabetes, asthma and disorders of sexual glands
	Obesity of thighs and calves
	Preparatory posture for Prāṇāyāma

MAKARĀSANA

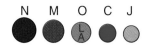

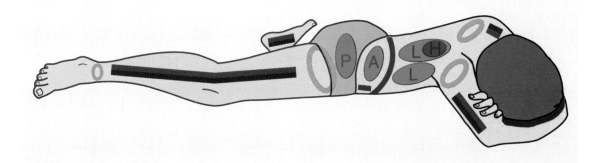

MAKARĀSANA

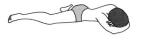

मकरासन

Crocodile Pose

Main Steps	Lie on belly with chin on floor and crossed forearms above the head.
	Inhale, raise chest, bring arms in line with shoulders, and place forehead on the crossed forearms.
	Keep legs astride as far as possible, with inner borders of feet touching the floor.
	Keep chest above ground and abdomen in full contact with the floor.
	Do abdominal breathing, with abdomen moving towards the floor during inhalation and away from the floor during exhalation.
	Exhale and return to original position.
	Keep face sideways on the floor and arms on the side of the thighs and breathe normally.
Benefits	Reduces stress and fatigue.
	Strengthens the diaphragm.
	Improves diaphragmatic breathing.
	Massages chest and abdominal organs: heart, lungs, stomach, liver, spleen, intestines and gall bladder.
	Tones the heart.
	Loosens shoulder, hip and ankle joints.
Indications	Stress related disorders: hypertension, peptic ulcer, colitis, diabetes and asthma
	General physical and mental fatigue
	Gastro-intestinal disorders: dyspepsia, peptic ulcer and constipation
	Respiratory disorders: chronic bronchitis and asthma
	Stiffness of shoulder, hip and ankle joints

PAWANMUKTĀSANA

O E S J F

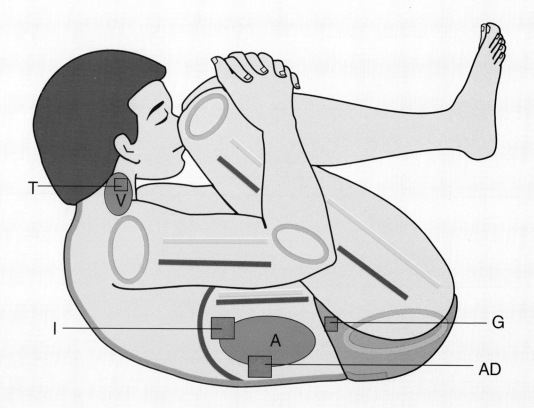

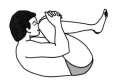

PAWANMUKTĀSANA

पवनमुक्तासन

Gas Releasing Pose

Main Steps	Lie on back with feet together.
	Exhale and bend both knees and hold shins down with locked hands or crossed forearms.
	Exhale and press thighs gently towards lower abdomen.
	Exhale and raise head up and touch forehead to knees.
	Maintain the pose and breathe normally.
	Inhale and return to original position.
	Note: if you have a sore back, use one pillow under the hips and another between the neck and shoulder blades to relieve strain on back.
Benefits	Massages abdominal organs: stomach and intestines.
	Massages endocrine glands: thyroid, parathyroids, islets of Langerhans, adrenals and gonads.
	Tones the spine.
	Loosens knee, hip, elbow and finger joints.
	Reduces obesity of abdomen, thighs and arms.
	Strengthens abdominal and neck muscles.
Indications	Digestive disorders: dyspepsia, flatulence, eructations, constipation and colitis
	Gallbladder, spleen and liver disorders
	Thyroid , parathyroid, and gonad disorders
	Diabetes
	Weak spine
	Arthritis
	Obesity of abdomen, thighs and arms
	Weak abdominal and neck muscles

ANANTĀSANA

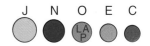

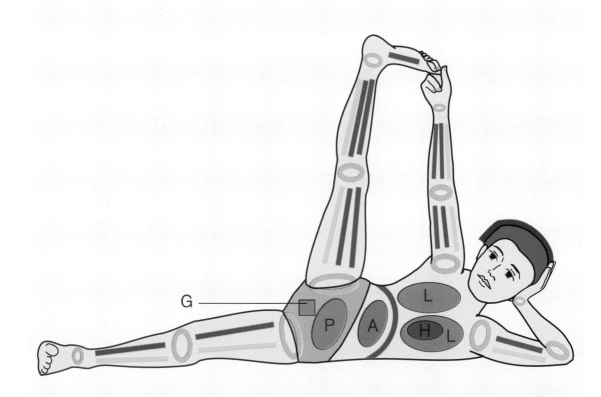

G

ANANTĀSANA

अनंतासन

God Vishnu's Resting Pose

Main Steps	Lie on back with feet together.
	Turn body to left and lie on left side with body in full contact with the floor.
	Extend left arm upwards, bend elbow, and rest portion of the head behind the left ear on the palm.
	Bend right knee and hold big toe with the fingers of the right hand.
	Exhale and extend right leg and arm vertically upwards simultaneously till knee and the elbow are locked.
	Maintain the pose and breathe normally.
	Exhale and return to original position.
	Repeat pose on opposite side.
Benefits	Strengthens joints of upper and lower extremities.
	Soothes mind and nerves.
	Stretches and relaxes nerves of legs and arms.
	Improves blood flow to pelvic organs and endocrine glands.
	Improves venous drainage from legs and arms.
	Tones the lungs and abdominal organs
Indications	Arthritis and sciatica
	Mental stress and strain
	Stress related disorders: hypertension, peptic ulcer, and colitis
	General physical and mental fatigue
	Genito-urinary disorders of uterus, urinary bladder, testes, ovaries and prostate
	Disorders of sex glands
	Oedema of legs or arms
	Menstrual disorders

SĀLAMBA SARVĀṄGĀSANA-I

EA ✓	MD	DI

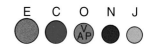

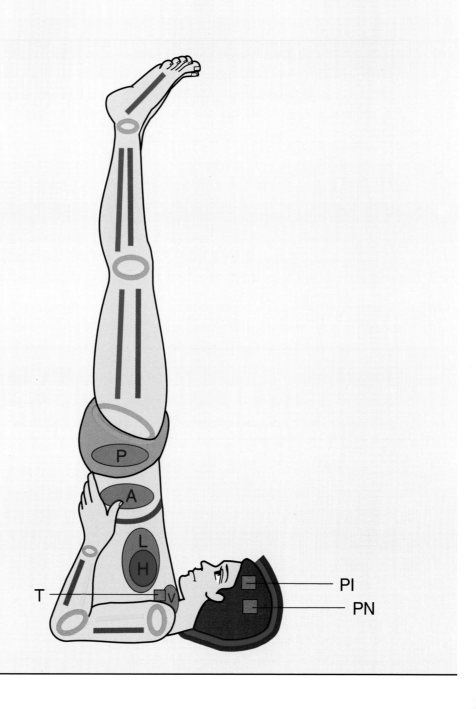

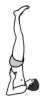

SĀLAMBA SARVĀṄGĀSANA - I

सालम्ब सर्वांगासन

Shoulder Stand

Main Steps	Lie on back with feet together and palms close to the body facing the floor.
	Bend the knees and rest thighs on the lower abdomen.
	Exhale and lift hips and thighs to 60° and support them with the palms and fingers by bending arms at the elbows.
	Exhale and lift trunk and thighs to a vertical position supporting the back with palms.
	Slide palms down on the back towards the head till chest touches chin.
	Straighten the legs and point toes upward.
	Maintain the pose and breathe normally.
	Exhale and slide down to original position.
	Caution: Refer to general instruction (Pg. xiii) for contra-indications.
Benefits	Improves blood flow to pituitary, pineal, thyroid and parathyroid glands.
	Improves blood flow to head, neck and brain.
	Improves blood flow to all the sense organs: eyes, nose, ears, tongue and the skin of the face.
	Reduces swelling of feet and legs and pelvic congestion.
	Replaces sagging abdominal organs back to their position.
	Strengthens joints of upper extremities.
	Reduces mental and physical fatigue.
Indications	Pituitary, thyroid, parathyroid and gonad disorders
	Insomnia, poor memory and concentration
	Oedema of feet and legs, and piles
	Mild giddiness
	Gastro-intestinal disorders of stomach and intestines
	Genito-urinary disorders of urinary bladder, uterus and prostate
	Physical and mental fatigue
	Weak joints of upper extremities
	As a preparatory posture to Śīrṣāsana

ADHO MUKHA ŚVĀNĀSANA

EA	MD ✓	DI

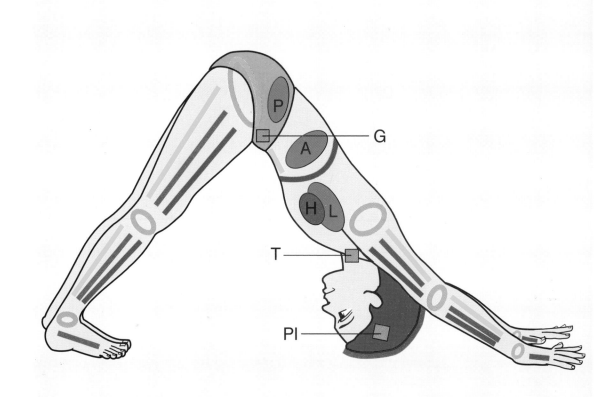

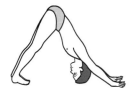

ADHO MUKHA ŚVĀNĀSANA

अधो मुख श्वानासन

Dog, Face Down Pose

Main Steps	Lie on your belly with forehead on the floor, feet one foot apart, and hands close to your shoulder with the elbows bent vertically.
	Raise the hips up by straightening the arms and bending the knees.
	Lift the hips up still higher by straightening the knees, allowing the tail bone to become the highest point.
	Move shoulders and chest downwards and backwards towards thighs.
	Stretch the legs by allowing the heels to move downward maintaining the tail bone at the same height.
	Allow the head to relax and to rest on the floor or on one or two folded blankets as required.
	Maintain the pose and breathe normally.
	Exhale and return to original position by retracing the steps in the reverse order.
	Keep face sideways on the floor, arms on the side of the thighs and breathe normally.
Benefits	Improves blood flow to brain, head, neck, fingers and toes.
	Improves blood flow to pituitary, pineal, thyroid and parathyroid glands and reduces congestion in gonads.
	Reduces congestion in pelvic and abdominal organs.
	Drains the lungs.
	Strengthens muscles and joints of upper and lower extremities.
	Reduces fat in upper and lower extremities.
	Increases stamina.
	Improves memory, concentration, intellect and creativity.
Indications	Hair loss and insomnia
	Thyroid, parathyroid and sexual disorders
	Respiratory disorders: chronic bronchitis
	Genito-urinary and menstrual disorders
	Arthritis
	Weakness or obesity of arms and legs
	Stress related disorders (with head resting on support)
	Poor memory and concentration

PRASĀRITA PĀDOTTĀNĀSANA

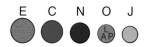

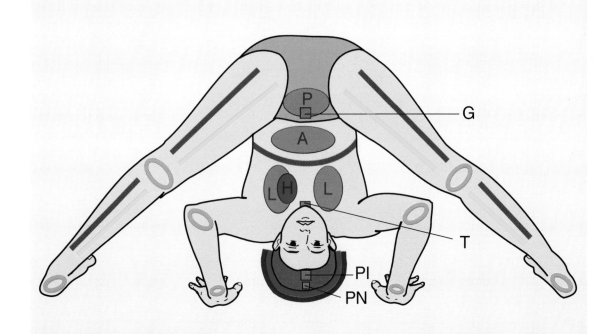

PRASĀRITA PĀDOTTĀNĀSANA

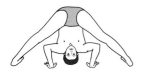

प्रसारित पादोत्तानासन

Wide Legs Stretching Pose

Main Steps	Stand in Tāḍāsana (p. 1).
	Jump 4 feet apart and place hands on waist.
	Exhale, bend forwards with neck extended and back concave, and place palms on floor between the feet.
	Exhale and bend elbows to allow head to rest on the floor between the two palms.
	Note: If you find it hard to place head on floor, spread your legs to the maximum or use folded blankets to rest the head.
	Keep medial arches of feet raised.
	Maintain the pose and breathe normally.
	Inhale and return to original position.
Benefits	Improves blood flow to head, neck and trunk.
	Improves blood flow to pituitary, pineal, thyroid, parathyroid and thymus glands.
	Reduces mental and physical fatigue.
	Strengthens legs and reduces fat around thighs.
	Strengthens ankle and wrist joints.
	Reduces congestion in abdominal and pelvic organs and gonads.
	Drains out secretions from lungs.
Indications	Migraine, insomnia, lack of concentration, poor memory and mental fatigue
	Pituitary, thyroid and parathyroid disorders
	Physical or mental fatigue (with head resting on support)
	Weakness of legs and fat around the thighs
	Weakness of ankle, wrist and elbow joints
	Menstrual disorders
	Disorders of sex glands
	Pelvic organ disorders of urinary bladder, uterus and prostate

ARDHA CHANDRĀSANA

EA	MD	DI ✓

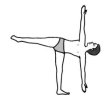

ARDHA CHANDRĀSANA

अर्ध चन्द्रासन

Half Moon Pose

Main Steps	Do Trikoṇāsana (p. 9).
	Bend left knee, drag right foot forwards and put left hand on the floor, one foot away and slightly outside or in line with the trunk line.
	Exhale and straighten left leg and raise right leg simultaneously to bring it in line with the trunk, with the palms of both hands and the toes of right foot pointing forwards.
	Turn head upwards and gaze at right thumb balancing the body on the left hand and leg.
	Maintain the pose and breathe normally.
	Exhale and return to the original pose by retracing the steps in the reverse order.
	Repeat the pose on the opposite side.
Benefits	Reduces congestion in abdominal and pelvic organs.
	Drains phlegm (thick mucous) from lungs.
	Improves balance and poise.
	Strengthens inner ears and eyes.
	Improves circulation to the head, neck, hypothalamus and endocrine glands in brain and neck.
	Helps venous drainage from extremities.
	Tones spine.
	Strengthens legs, knees and hip joints.
	Reduces fat around thighs.
Indications	Genito-urinary disorders of urinary bladder and uterus
	Gastro-intestinal disorders: indigestion and dyspepsia
	Chronic bronchitis
	Mild giddiness
	Poor memory, concentration and eye-sight
	Insomnia and falling hair
	Endocrine disorders of pituitary, thyroid and parathyroid glands
	Arthritis
	Stiffness of spine
	Obesity of thighs and weakness of legs

SETU BANDHA SARVĀṄGĀSANA

S O N E J

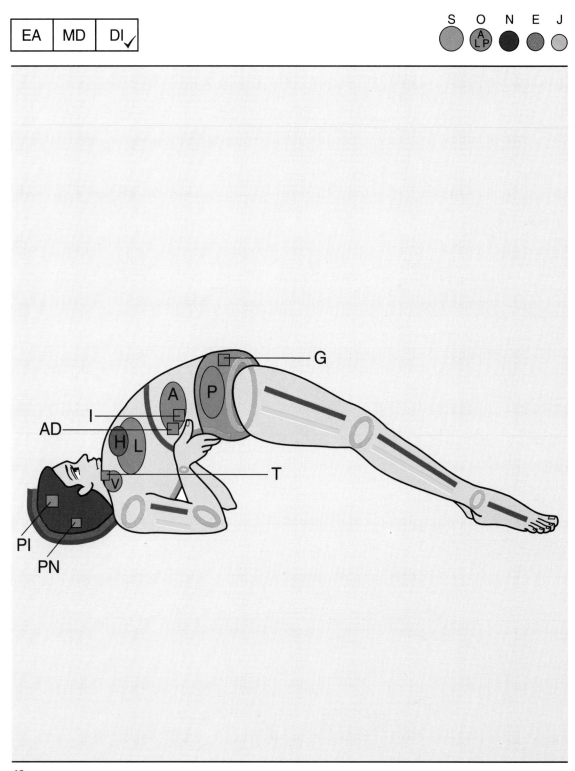

SETU BANDHA SARVĀṄGĀSANA

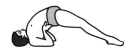

सेतुबन्ध सर्वांगासन

Bridge Pose

Main Steps	Do Sarvāṅgāsana (p. 53).
	Bend the knees and allow trunk to fall to the floor over the wrists, firmly supporting the lower dorsal spine with the palms.
	Straighten the legs slowly one at a time and keep feet together.
	Maintain the pose and breathe normally.
	Exhale and gradually lower the body to a lying position and breathe normally.
	Note: If you cannot do it independently, use a long bench to support the hips and legs.
Benefits	Tones lumbo-dorsal spine.
	Broadens chest and expands lungs.
	Massages abdominal and pelvic organs.
	Improves blood flow to neck, brain and hypothalamus.
	Soothes nervous system and mind.
	Increases blood supply and massages thyroid and parathyroid glands.
	Reduces fat around thighs and arms.
	Strengthens arms, wrists and ankles.
	Reduces congestion of gonads.
Indications	Spondylitis and backaches
	Respiratory disorders: asthma and bronchitis
	Gastro-intestinal and pelvic organ disorders
	General apathy and mental depression
	Insomnia, poor memory, lack of concentration
	Thyroid and parathyroid dysfunction
	Disorders of sex glands
	Weakness of arms, wrists and ankles
	Fat around thighs and arms

HALĀSANA

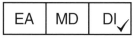

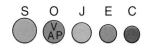

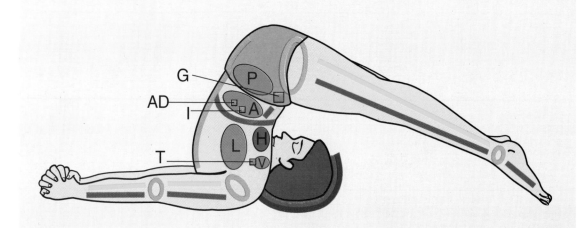

HALĀSANA

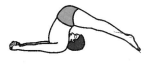

हलासन

Plough Pose

Main Steps	Do Sālamba Sarvāṅgāsana (p. 53).
	Release chin lock and lower trunk and legs gently to the floor on the head side, bringing arms upward under the legs at the same time.
	Note: In case the feet do not reach the floor, do half Halāsana with the legs resting on a bench or a stool of the appropriate height.
	Raise trunk further up to a vertical level by contracting muscles of the thighs, and by placing hands in middle of back and lifting it.
	Release hands and stretch them back in a direction opposite to that of the legs.
	Maintain the pose and breathe normally.
	Exhale and return to Sarvāṅgāsana and then slowly lower the trunk and the legs to the floor.

Benefits	Reduces stiffness of shoulders and back.
	Massages abdominal organs.
	Relieves congestion from pelvic organs and gonads.
	Tones endocrine glands: pituitary, pineal, thyroid, parathyroid, adrenals and islets of Langerhans.
	Quietens and rejuvenates the mind.
	Loosens joints of upper and lower extremities.
	Improves circulation to brain, hypothalamus, head and neck.

Indications	Stiffness of back and shoulders
	Gastro-intestinal disorders of liver, spleen and pancreas
	Genito-urinary disorders of urinary bladder, prostate, ovaries and testes
	Stress related diseases: diabetes, asthma, and colitis
	Pituitary, thyroid and parathyroid disorders
	Diabetes
	Mental tension, anxiety and depression

SĀLAMBA ŚĪRṢĀSANA

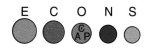

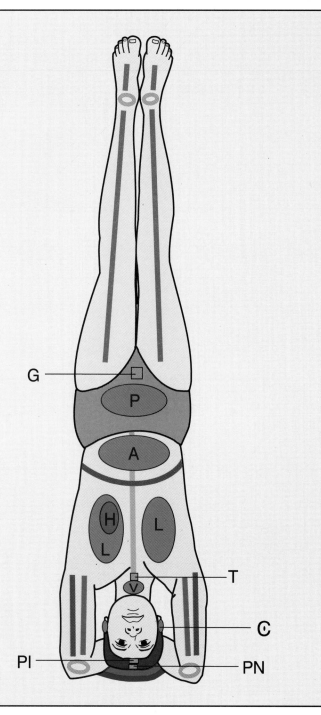

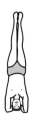

SĀLAMBA ŚĪRṢĀSANA

सालंब शीर्षासन

Head Stand

Main Steps	Kneel behind a folded blanket, bend forwards, place arms on blanket parallel to each other and in line with the shoulders.
	Without shifting elbows, bring hands close to each other and interlock fingers to form a cup, resting on the inner borders of the palms.
	Place crown of head on blanket so that back of head fits snugly in the cup of the palms.
	Raise knees and hips up and walk in towards trunk, allowing it to become as vertical as possible.
	Exhale and with a gentle swing, lift feet off the floor with bent knees.
	Straighten thighs first, followed by the legs, and balance body on crown of head keeping legs, trunk, neck and head in one line.
	Maintain the pose and breathe normally.
	Exhale and return to original position.
	Caution: Refer to general instructions (p. xiii) for contra-indications.
Benefits	Improves blood flow to pituitary, pineal, thyroid and parathyroid glands.
	Removes congestion from gonads.
	Improves blood flow to brain, hypothalamus, head and neck.
	Improves balance, concentration, confidence, will power and creativity.
	Strengthens inner ears and eyes.
	Helps venous drainage from lower extremities and pelvis.
	Replaces sagging abdominal organs to their original place.
	Drains secretions from lungs and improves ventilation.
	Improves alignment of back and spine.
Indications	Endocrine disorders and poor body immunity
	Weak eyes, inner ears and other senses
	Poor memory, intelligence, concentration and will power
	Baldness, insomnia and migraine
	Varicose veins, oedema of feet and piles
	Visceroptosis, inguinal hernias, constipation and uterine prolapse
	Poor lung power, chronic coughs, colds, tonsillitis and halitosis (foul breath)
	Physical or mental fatigue
	Stiffness of back and spine

BHUJAṄGĀSANA

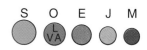

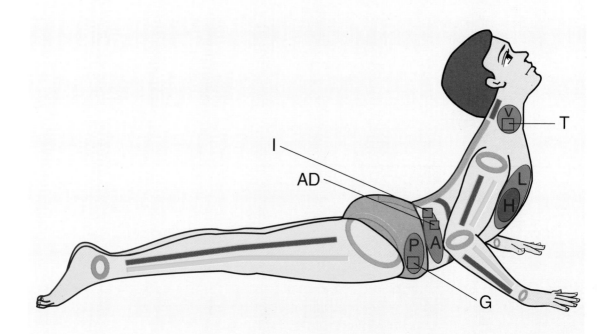

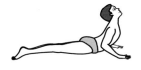

BHUJAṄGĀSANA

भुजंगासन

Cobra Pose

Main Steps	Lie on belly with forehead on floor and arms close to the chest.
	Bend elbows and bring hands close to the shoulders, with fingers spread out.
	Inhale and raise head, neck, chest and upper belly off the floor, keeping lower belly and pubis on the floor.
	Keep remaining portion of the body in close contact with the floor.
	Keep hips, thighs and knees firm and contracted.
	Extend neck fully, look towards the heart and brace shoulders backward.
	Maintain the pose and breathe normally.
	Exhale and return to original position.
Benefits	Strengthens complete spine, posterior spinal muscles and ligaments.
	Tones larynx, heart and neck muscles.
	Broadens the chest.
	Stimulates abdominal and pelvic organs.
	Stimulates thyroid, parathyroid, adrenal glands and islets of Langerhans.
	Strengthens joints of upper extremities.
	Tones hip and thigh muscles.
Indications	Cervical and thoracic spondylitis
	High and mid-backaches
	Early slipped discs and sciatica
	Voice disorders
	Asthma and bronchitis
	Abdominal and pelvic organ disorders
	Thyroid and parathyroid disorders, diabetes and asthma
	Arthritis of upper extremity joints

ŚALABHĀSANA

S O E M J

ŚALABHĀSANA

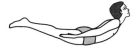

शलभासन

Locust Pose

Main Steps	Lie on belly with forehead on the floor, feet together with toes pointing backwards, and arms close to body, palms facing upwards.
	Inhale and raise head, chest and thighs up simultaneously, as high as possible along with the arms pointing towards the toes at shoulder level without bending knees.
	Body should be resting only on the abdomen.
	Contract hip muscles and close the anus.
	Keep elbows and knees locked.
	Maintain the pose and breathe normally.
	Exhale and return to original position.
	Keep face sideways on the floor, arms on side of thighs and breathe normally.
	Note: In persons who have backache and the pose hurts the back more, avoid the pose till back gains strength.
Benefits	Tones complete spine.
	Tones abdominal organs and heart.
	Expands chest and lungs.
	Tones thyroid, parathyroid, adrenals, islets of Langerhans and gonads.
	Strengthens muscles of back, thighs, arms, neck and front of abdomen.
	Strengthens all joints of upper and lower extremities.
Indications	Cervical, thoracic and lumbar spondylitis
	Upper, mid and low backaches
	Gastro-intestinal disorders of liver, spleen, gall bladder and stomach
	Asthma, bronchitis and emphysema
	Thyroid and parathyroid disorders
	Diabetes and disorders of sex glands
	Protruding and weak abdomen
	Arthritis

ŪRDHVA MUKHA ŚVĀNĀSANA

S   O E J M

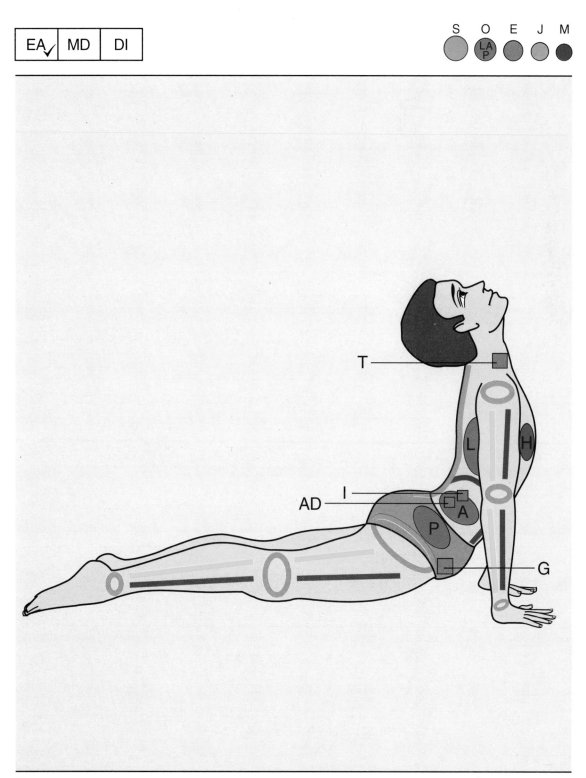

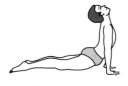

ŪRDHVA MUKHA ŚVĀNĀSANA

ऊर्ध्व मुख श्वानासन

Dog, Face Upward Pose

Main Steps	Lie on the belly with forehead on the floor, feet one foot apart and hands close to the waist, with elbows bent.
	Raise and extend head, neck, chest, abdomen, thighs, knees and legs completely by gradually straightening the arms.
	Maintain the pose by resting only on the palms and extended toes.
	Push chest forwards and tighten the hip muscles.
	Maintain the pose and breathe normally.
	Exhale and return to original position.
	Keep face sideways on the floor, arms on the side of the thighs, palms facing upwards and breathe normally.
Benefits	Tones complete spine and heart.
	Expands chest and lungs.
	Massages abdominal and pelvic organs.
	Tones thyroid, adrenals, islets of Langerhans and gonads.
	Strengthens all the joints and muscles of upper and lower extremities.
	Reduces fat around the abdomen, arms and legs.
Indications	Spondylitis
	Respiratory diseases: asthma, chronic bronchitis and emphysema
	Gastro-intestinal disorders of liver, spleen, stomach and intestines
	Genito-urinary disorders of urinary bladder, uterus and prostate
	Thyroid, adrenal and gonad disorders
	Diabetes
	Arthritis
	Obesity of abdomen, arms or legs

MATSYĀSANA

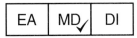

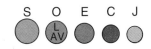

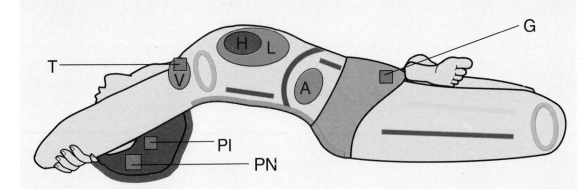

MATSYĀSANA

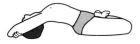

मत्स्यासन

Fish Pose

Main Steps	Sit in Padmāsana (p. 29).
	Exhale and arch the back to lower the head, neck and back, till crown of the head rests on the floor.
	Hold the feet in your hands and increase the arch of the back and the chest.
	Bend the arms, hold elbows and rest the arms behind the head.
	Maintain the pose and breathe normally.
	Exhale and return to original pose.
Benefits	Tones cervical and thoracic spine.
	Expands chest and lungs.
	Massages thyroid and parathyroid glands.
	Tones larynx and heart.
	Relieves pelvic congestion.
	Loosens shoulder and ankle joints.
Indications	Cervical and thoracic spondylitis
	Respiratory disorders: asthma, bronchitis
	Thyroid and parathyroid disorders
	Voice disorders
	Menstrual disorders
	Stiffness of shoulder and ankle joints
	Counter pose to Sarvāṅgāsana (p. 53)

UȘTRĂSANA

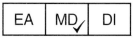

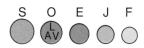

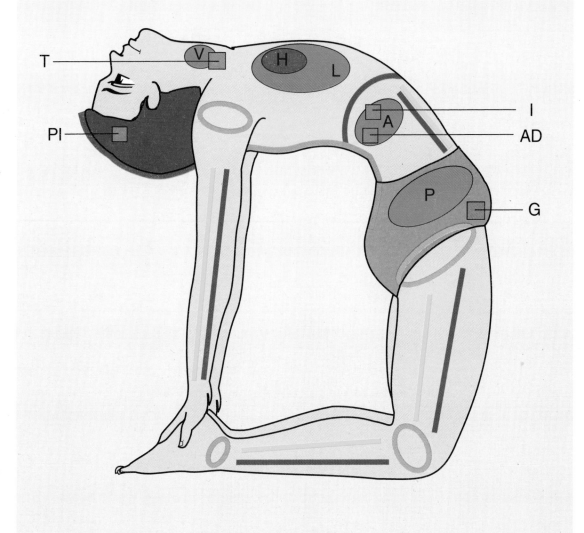

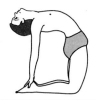

UṢṬRĀSANA

उष्ट्रासन

Camel Pose

Main Steps	Kneel with thighs and trunk erect, and hands on hips.

Main Steps

Kneel with thighs and trunk erect, and hands on hips.

Exhale and arch backwards.

Arch more by sliding hands down on back of thighs extending the head and neck backwards.

Exhale and release hands one at a time to hold the heels.

Press heels with hands to push spine towards thighs which are kept erect.

Maintain the pose and breathe normally.

Return to original position by replacing hands on thighs and walk up with the hands to allow head, neck, trunk and spine to come in one line.

Bend knees and sit in Vīrāsana pose (p. 25).

Bend forwards to rest forehead on the floor in Adho Mukha Vīrāsana pose (p. 27).

Benefits

Tones complete spine.

Broadens chest and expands lungs.

Tones larynx, heart and neck muscles.

Tones abdominal and pelvic organs.

Stimulates all endocrine glands.

Strengthens shoulder and hip joints.

Reduces fat around thighs.

Indications

Spondylitis of cervical, thoracic and lumbar spine

Respiratory disorders: asthma, bronchitis and emphysema

Voice disorders

Gastro-intestinal disorders: dyspepsia, constipation, colitis, liver and gall-bladder disorders

Genito-urinary disorders of kidney, urinary bladder, ovaries, testes and prostate

Thyroid and parathyroid disorders

Diabetes

Stiffness of shoulder and hip joints

Obesity of thighs

DHANURĀSANA

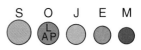

EA	MD ✓	DI

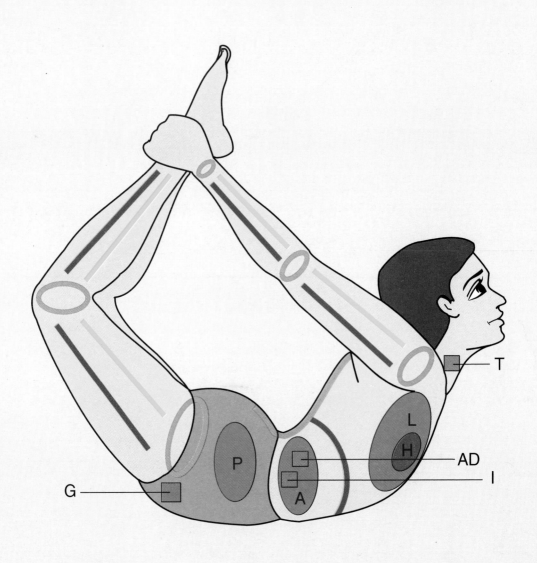

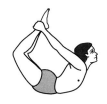

DHANURĀSANA

धनुरासन

Bow Pose

Main Steps	Lie down on belly with forehead on the floor, arms on side of thighs and feet slightly apart.
	Bend knees and hold ankles with outstretched hands.
	Exhale completely and lift knees and chest up simultaneously by pulling on the shins with the arms.
	Raise thighs and chest further upwards by allowing the feet to move towards the ceiling and allowing the head to be extended back as far as possible.
	Approximate ankles, knees and thighs.
	Maintain the pose and breathe normally.
	Exhale and return to original position.
Benefits	Brings elasticity and flexibility to spine.
	Massages abdominal and pelvic organs.
	Expands chest and lungs.
	Tones heart, adrenals, islets of Langerhans and gonads.
	Strengthens upper and lower extremities.
	Loosens joints of extremities.
	Reduces fat around the waist, thighs and arms.
	Strengthens neck.
Indications	Backaches and mild disc problems
	Cervical, thoracic and lumbar spondylitis
	Gastro-intestinal disorders of liver, spleen and intestines
	Respiratory disorders: chronic bronchitis and asthma
	Genito-urinary disorders of kidneys, urinary bladder, uterus, sex glands and prostate
	Diabetes, asthma and sexual disorders
	Weakness of upper and lower extremities
	Obesity around waist, thighs and arms

ŪRDHVA DHANURĀSANA

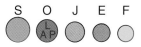

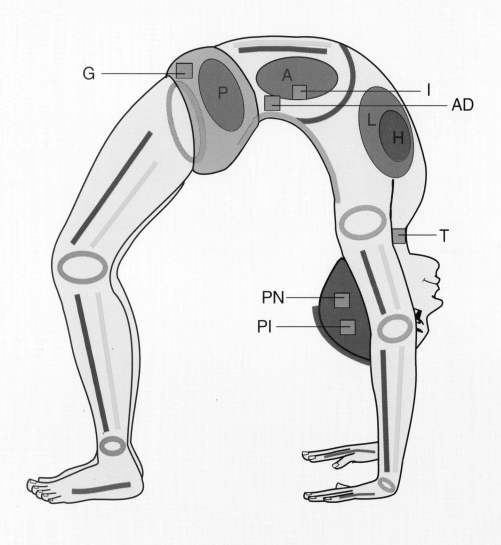

ŪRDHVA DHANURĀSANA

ऊर्ध्व धनुरासन

Upward Bow Pose

Main Steps

Lie on back with feet 6 inches apart.

Bend knees and bring feet close to the thighs.

Take arms over the head and place them close to the shoulders with elbows bent and fingers pointing towards feet.

Exhale and raise trunk and chest, by putting pressure of hands and feet on the ground and opening up elbows and knees partially.

Place crown of head on ground by extending the neck.

Exhale and raise head from the floor and take trunk still higher by straightening the arms and raising the thighs and abdomen as high as possible.

Keep palms and soles of feet firmly on the floor.

Maintain the pose and breathe normally.

Exhale, lower the body gently to the floor and breathe normally.

Benefits

Strengthens complete spine.

Tones heart and abdominal organs.

Strengthens all joints.

Stretches and strengthens muscles of frontal abdomen, extremities and the back.

Expands chest and lungs.

Tones all endocrine glands.

Reduces fat around abdomen and extremities.

Indications

Spondylitis, backaches, early disc problems and sciatica

Gastro-intestinal disorders of liver, pancreas, spleen, stomach and gall bladder

Weakness of muscles and joints of upper and lower extremities

Respiratory disorders: asthma and bronchitis

Endocrinological disorders: diabetes, thyroid and disorders of the sex glands

Genito-urinary disorders of kidneys, urinary bladder, uterus and prostate

Obesity

EKA PĀDA RĀJAKAPOTĀSANA - I

S O E J M

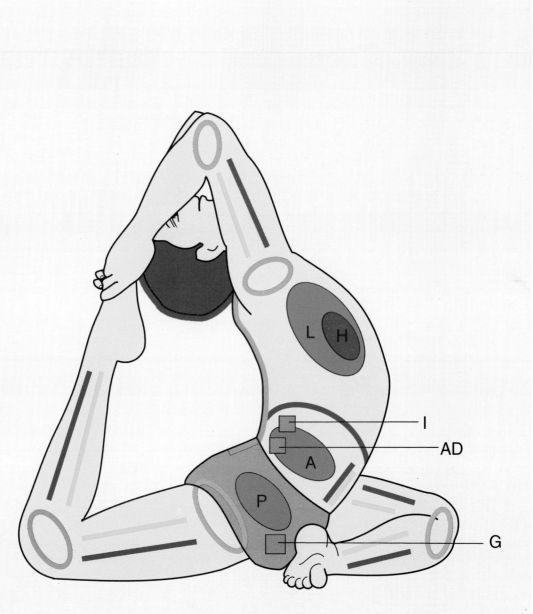

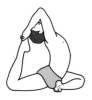

EKA PĀDA RĀJAKAPOTĀSANA-I

एक पाद राजकपोतासन

Pigeon Pose

Main Steps	Sit with legs straight.
	Bend left knee parallel to the floor and touch heel to right groin.
	Take right leg back and stretch it straight with toes pointing backwards.
	Put hands on waist and throw the head back.
	Place hands on floor, bend the right knee and bring foot close to the head.
	Exhale and take both arms, one at a time over the head, to hold the right foot.
	Maintain the pose and breathe normally.
	Exhale and return to original position by retracing the steps in the reverse order.
	Repeat the pose on opposite side.
Benefits	Rejuvenates lower spine.
	Broadens chest and expands lungs.
	Strengthens larynx.
	Tones all endocrine glands, abdominal and pelvic organs.
	Strengthens all joints.
	Strengthens neck, shoulders, groins and thighs.
Indications	Spondylitis and lumbo-sacral backache
	Gastro-intestinal and pelvic organ disorders
	Asthma and bronchitis
	Voice disorders
	Thyroid and parathyroid disorders
	Diabetes and disorders of sex glands
	Arthritis
	Weak neck, shoulders and thighs
	Obesity of abdomen and thighs

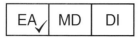

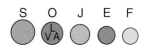

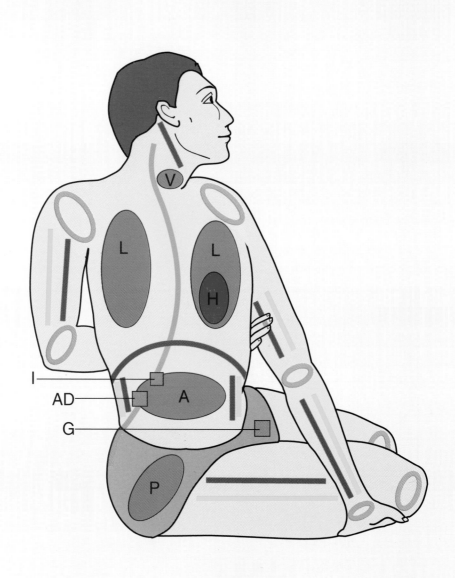

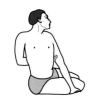

BHĀRADVĀJĀSANA-I

भारद्वाजासन

Bharadvaj's Pose

Main Steps	Sit with feet straight and spine erect.
	Bend both knees so that they point to the right and the feet to the left, and raise the left arm up.
	Exhale and twist trunk towards the right, bring down and push left hand under right thigh, with palm facing the floor.
	Take right hand behind back, and hold left arm.
	Look over the left shoulder.
	Maintain the pose and breathe normally.
	Inhale and return to original position by retracing the steps in the reverse order.
	Repeat pose on the opposite side.
Benefits	Tones complete spine.
	Massages abdominal organs, especially kidneys.
	Opens chest and lungs.
	Loosens all joints.
	Massages endocrine glands: adrenals, islets of Langerhans and gonads.
	Narrows the waist.
	Tones neck muscles, larynx and heart.
Indications	Lumbago and spondylitis
	Genito-urinary disorders of ovaries, testes, prostate, urinary bladder and kidney.
	Gastro-intestinal disorders of liver, spleen, intestines and pancreas
	Respiratory disorders: chronic bronchitis, asthma and bronchiectasis
	Arthritis
	Diabetes
	Obesity
	Voice disorders

MARĪCYĀSANA - I

EA ✓	MD	DI

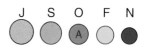

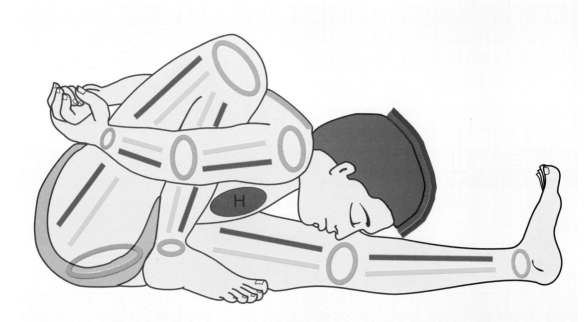

MARĪCYĀSANA-I

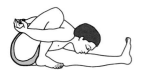

मरीच्यासन

Sage Marich's Pose

Main Steps	Sit with legs straight and spine erect.
	Bend right knee vertically and place right heel close to right thigh.
	Take right arm over the right knee to hold the left toes and twist towards the left.
	Take left hand behind the back, and revolve the right hand around the right shin, to hold left hand behind the back.
	Bring trunk in line with the left thigh and bend forwards to touch chin to left thigh or shin.
	Maintain the pose and breathe normally.
	Inhale and return to original position by retracing the steps in the reverse order.
	Repeat pose on opposite side.
Benefits	Loosens all joints.
	Reduces stiffness in the spine.
	Tones and massages abdominal organs and endocrine glands.
	Reduces fat around thighs and abdomen.
	Reduces physical and mental stress.
Indications	Arthritis
	Stiffness of spine
	Gastro-intestinal disorders of stomach, intestines, liver, spleen and pancreas
	Obesity of abdomen and thighs
	Mental and physical fatigue
	Diabetes

ARDHA MATSYENDRĀSANA-I

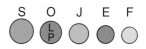

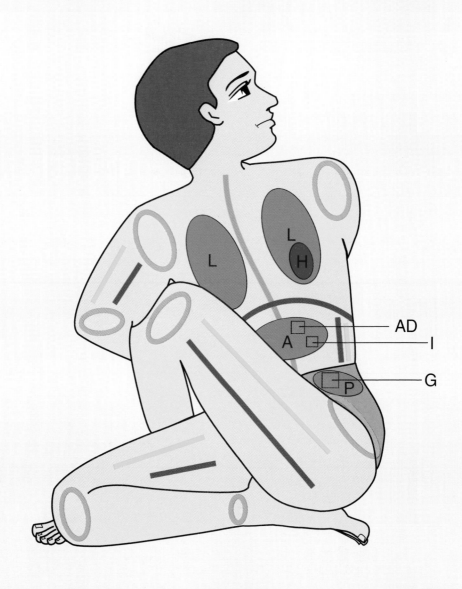

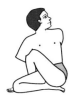

ARDHA MATSYENDRĀSANA-I

अर्ध मत्स्येन्द्रासन

Lord Matsyendra's Pose

Main Steps	Sit with legs stretched in front.
	Bend right knee parallel to the floor, raise the hips, place foot horizontally under them and sit over it.
	Bend left knee vertically and place foot on outer side of right thigh with shin perpendicular to floor.
	Exhale and twist 90° to left, and bring right armpit over the left knee.
	Exhale and twist right arm around the left knee, and place it behind the back.
	Exhale and take left arm back, and grip the opposite hand.
	Turn head to left or right, and gaze at centre of eyebrows or over the shoulder.
	Maintain the pose and breathe normally.
	Exhale and return to original position by retracing the steps in a reverse order.
	Repeat the pose sitting on the left foot and twisting to the right.
Benefits	Tones complete spine.
	Massages abdominal and pelvic organs, especially the kidneys.
	Loosens all joints.
	Tones gonads and adrenal glands.
	Reduces fat around thighs, arms and waist.
Indications	Spondylitis and backaches
	Genito-urinary disorders of kidney, urinary bladder, uterus, ovary, testes and prostate
	Gastro-intestinal disorders of liver, spleen and pancreas
	Arthritis
	Obesity of thighs, arms and waist

JĀNU ŚĪRṢĀSANA

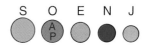

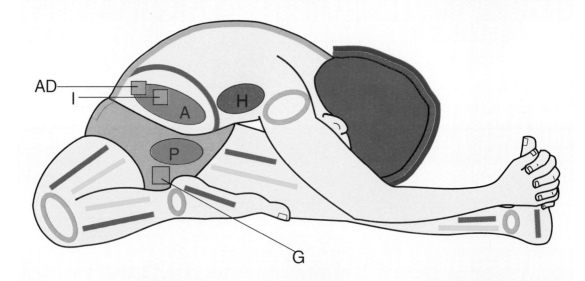

JĀNU ŚĪRṢĀSANA

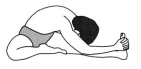

जानु शीर्षासन

Head Knee Pose

Main Steps	Sit with legs straight and back erect.
	Bend right knee moving it to the right along the floor and place foot against left thigh as high as possible.
	Allow right knee to go backwards as much as possible to form an obtuse angle between left and right thighs.
	Twist towards left with back straight to bring trunk in line with left leg.
	Inhale and raise arms up.
	Exhale and bend trunk and arms forward to hold sides of foot of extended leg.
	Bend and widen elbows to allow trunk to move forwards.
	Allow head to rest on leg and keep extended chest on thigh.
	Maintain pose and breathe normally.
	Inhale and return to original position by retracing the steps in the reverse order.
	Repeat pose with opposite leg straight.
Benefits	Tones complete spine.
	Tones abdominal organs.
	Relieves congestion in pelvic organs: prostate and gonads.
	Improve blood flow to pituitary, pineal, thyroid and parathyroid.
	Tones adrenals and islets of Langerhans.
	Soothes nerves and mind.
	Reduces stress and strain.
	Loosens joints of upper and lower extremities.
	Narrows the waist.
Indications	Rigid and stiff spine
	Indigestion and constipation
	Liver, spleen and kidney disorders
	Menstrual and sex gland disorders
	Stress related diseases: hypertension, peptic ulcer, colitis, asthma, diabetes (with head resting on support)
	Mental or physical fatigue
	Arthritis
	Broad waist

PAŚCIMOTTĀNĀSANA

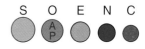

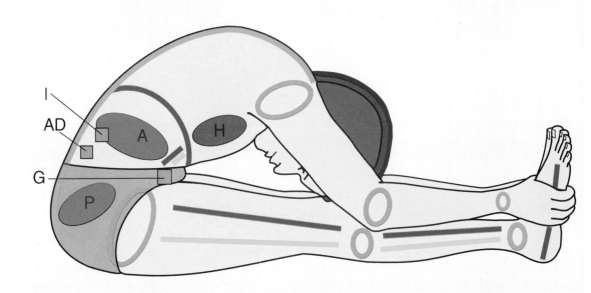

PAŚCIMOTTĀNĀSANA

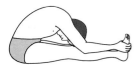

पश्चिमोत्तानासन

Back Spine Stretching Pose

Main Steps	Sit with legs straight and back erect.
	Exhale and lean forwards, and extending the arms from the shoulders hold the toes.
	Exhale, bend forwards more by widening the elbows outwards.
	Bend and extend trunk further forwards and downwards from the hips towards legs, placing forehead on knees or legs or on support if unable to rest head on knees or legs.
	Hold toes or outer borders of feet in the middle of the soles.
	Maintain the pose and breathe normally.
	Inhale and return to original position by retracing the steps in a reverse order.
Benefits	Tones complete spine.
	Massages abdominal and pelvic organs.
	Improves digestion.
	Tones endocrine glands: adrenals, islets of Langerhans and gonads.
	Removes mental and physical fatigue.
	Improves circulation to head and neck.
	Loosens all joints.
Indications	Backaches and arthritis
	Gastro-intestinal disorders: constipation and dyspepsia
	Diabetes, asthma and disorders of the sex glands
	Menstrual disorders
	Stress related disorders: asthma, diabetes, peptic ulcer and colitis (with head resting on support)
	Mental and physical fatigue

YOGA MUDRĀ

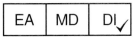

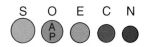

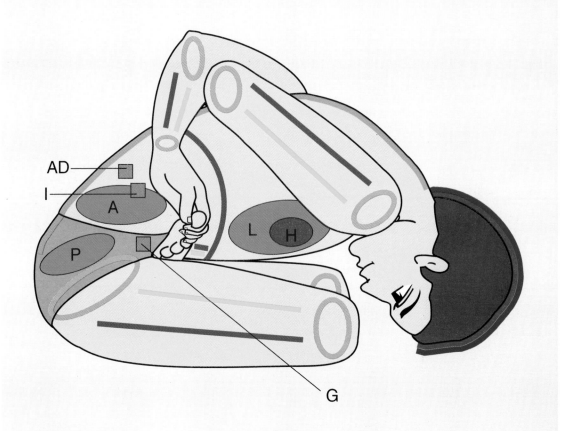

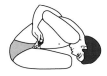

YOGA MUDRĀ

योग मुद्रा

Main Steps	Sit in Padmāsana (p. 29).

Take hands back and hold toes of same foot from behind.

Exhale and bend trunk forward and downward with a concave back.

Bring head gently to the floor.

Maintain the pose and breathe normally.

Inhale and return to original pose.

Repeat pose with opposite leg on top.

Benefits

Tones spine.

Massages abdominal organs.

Tones pelvic organs: urinary bladder, colon, rectum, prostate, and uterus.

Massages endocrine glands: islets of Langerhans, adrenals and gonads.

Increases blood flow to head and neck.

Loosens ankle, knee, hip and shoulder joints.

Reduces mental stress.

Indications

Stiffness of spine

Gastro-intestinal disorders: dyspepsia, colitis and constipation

Liver and spleen disorders

Genito-urinary disorders of urinary bladder, ovary and prostate

Diabetes and asthma

Menstrual disorders

General tiredness and fatigue

Mental stress and strain (with head resting on support)

ŚAVĀSANA

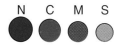

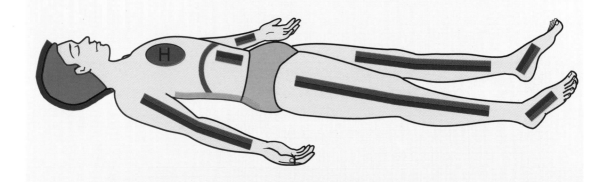

ŚAVĀSANA

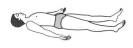

शवासन

Corpse Pose

Main Steps	Lie on back with centre of forehead, chin, sternum, navel and pubis in one line.
	Keep arms slightly away from side of body, palms facing upwards.
	Keep heels one foot apart with toes away from each other.
	Close eyes and consciously relax each and every part of the body including the mind by autosuggestion.
	Breathe normally with full awareness.
	Make the breath smooth, soft and effortless.
	Keep mind passive and watch the breath without taking any active part in the breathing process.
	Allow mind to descend towards the heart with each inhalation and exhalation.
	During the āsana do not go to sleep and be fully aware of the breath and the relaxed state of the body and mind.
	Slowly be aware of all body parts and open the eyes gently.
Benefits	Reduces physical, mental and emotional stress, strain and fatigue of all kinds.
	Gives total relaxation to body
	Soothes nerves and mind.
	Reduces basal metabolic rate, pulse rate and blood pressure.
Indications	Physical and mental fatigue or tension
	Insomnia, anxiety, neurosis and phobias
	Stress related diseases: asthma, diabetes, peptic ulcer, colitis and angina pectoris
	High blood pressure, tachycardia and hyper-thyroidism

UJJĀYI PRĀNĀYĀMA

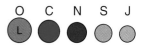

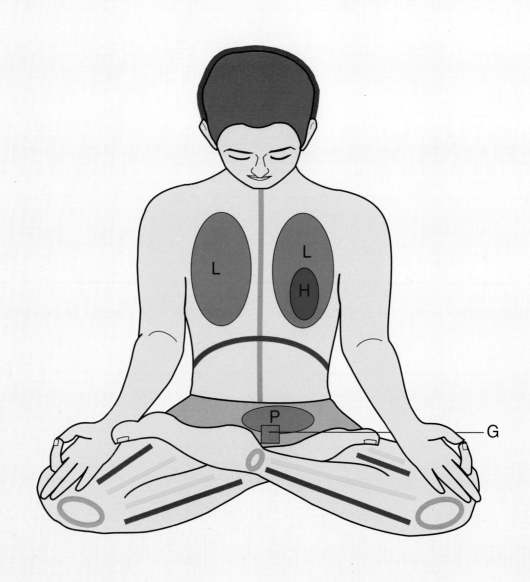

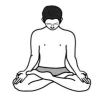

UJJĀYĪ PRĀṆĀYĀMA

उज्जायी प्राणायाम

Main Steps	Sit in Padmāsana with hands resting on the thighs with index fingers and thumbs forming a ring (gyana mudra).
	Keep the back absolutely erect and perpendicular to floor.
	Bring head down to rest in the notch between the collar bones (chin lock or Jalandhara bandha).
	Start Ujjāyī Prāṇāyāma as taught to you by your guru or yoga teacher **[without retentionof breath (kumbhaka) in cardio-respiratory disorders]**.
Benefits	Increases oxygenation of blood and tissues.
	Improves function of circulatory and respiratory systems.
	Improves function of all organs and systems.
	Expands chest and increases vital capacity of lungs.
	Soothes nervous system and mind.
	Pacifies gonads.
	Strengthens the spine.
	Other benefits of Padmāsana (p. 29).
Indications	Respiratory and cardio-vascular diseases **[without retention of breath (kumbhaka)]**
	Chronic coughs and colds
	Allergic conditions of the nose and chest
	Asthma
	Physical or mental fatigue
	To strengthen the spine

NĀDĪ ŚODHANA PRĀṆĀYĀMA

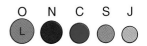

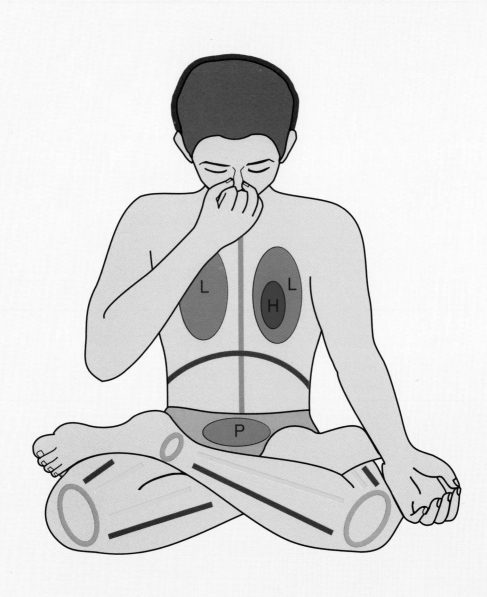

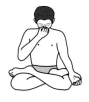

NĀDĪ ŚODHANA PRĀṆĀYĀMA

नाडी शोधन प्राणायाम

Alternate Nasal Breathing

Main Steps	Sit in Padmāsana (p. 29).
	Control nasal airway by thumb and fingers of right hand placed on either side of nose on tiny depressions just under lower edge of nasal bones.
	Minimum pressure and release from the thumb will control the right airway and from the ring and little fingers will control the left airway, with the index and middle fingers flexed in the palm.
	Bend head down towards the sternum into the chin lock position. (Jalandhra bandha)
	Start Nādī Śodhana Prāṇāyāma as taught to you by your guru or teacher.
	Breathing in through the left nostril and out though the right, followed by breathing in through the right and out through the left constitutes one cycle.
	Avoid retention of breath (kumbhaka) in problems of ears, eyes, heart, lungs and brain.
Benefits	Improves oxygenation of blood and tissues.
	Improves function of all organs and systems.
	Balances autonomic nervous system.
	Calms nerves and mind.
	Reduces stress and strain.
	Improves immune system.
	Stabilises cardio-respiratory system.
Indications	Respiratory disorders: asthma, bronchitis, respiratory tract infections, chronic coughs and colds (in all without retention of breath)
	Stress related disorders: vasomotor rhinitis, peptic ulcers, diabetes and colitis
	Physical or mental fatigue
	Cardiovascular disorders: angina pectoris, cardiac arrhythmias, hypertension **(in all without retention of breath or kumbhaka)**
	Convalescence from various diseases
	Insomnia, poor memory and concentration **(in all without retention of breath or kumbhaka)**

SAṆMUKHĪ MUDRĀ

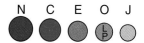

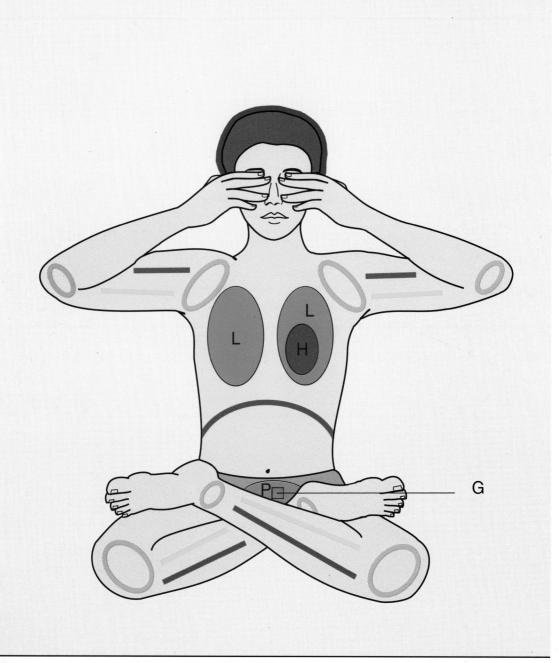

SAṆMUKHĪ MUDRĀ

षण्मुखी मुद्रा

Main Steps	Sit in Padmāsana (p. 29).
	Raise bent arms to shoulder level and close external ear canals with thumbs or by gentle pressure on the tragus.
	Place index and middle fingers gently on closed eyes which look upwards.
	Place ring fingers gently on the sides of the nostrils.
	Place little fingers on upper lip to feel flow of air through the nostrils.
	Breathe smoothly, gently and normally.
	Return to original position and gently open the eyes.
Benefits	Calms mind.
	Soothes nerves.
	Reduces blood pressure.
	Pacifies gonads.
	Increases blood flow to pelvic organs.
	Loosens joints of upper and lower extremities.
	Increases strength of arms.
Indications	Anxiety, mental tension and insomnia
	Nervousness and irritability
	High blood pressure
	Headaches, eye strain and tinnitus (noises in the ear)
	Genito-urinary disorders of urinary bladder, uterus and prostate
	Stiffness of lower extremity joints
	Disorder of sex glands

DHYĀNA

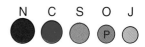

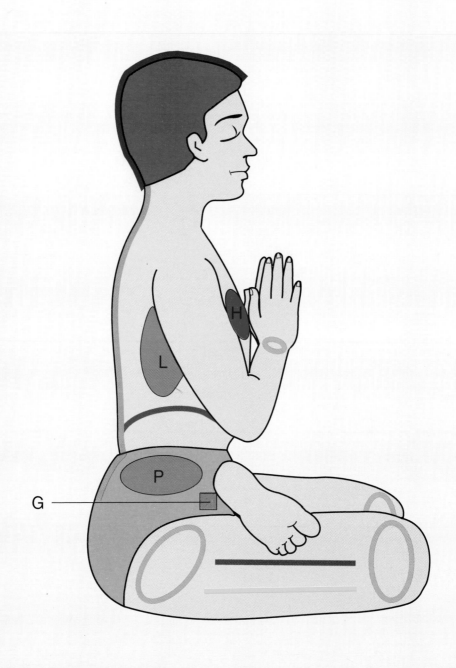

DHYĀNA

ध्यान

Meditation

Main Steps

Sit in Padmāsana (p. 29).

Join palms in prayer position in front of chest or keep them on the knees, with thumbs and index fingers forming a ring (gyana mudra).

Meditate as taught to you by your guru or yoga teacher.

Benefits

Quietens the mind.

Improves mental clarity and perception.

Stabilises nervous and cardio-vascular systems.

Lowers blood pressure and pulse rate.

Reduces metabolism.

Soothes gonads.

Indications

Mental stress and strain

High blood pressure

Hyperthyroidism and tachycardia

Poor memory and concentration

Insomnia

Stiffness of spine

Peptic ulcer

Sanskrit Pronunciations

a	as in around		ā	as in bath
i	as in blink		ī	as in bee
u	as in gut		ū	as in good

ś ṣ   as in shall

ṭ ḍ ṇ   pronounced with tongue curled back and hitting the upper palate

ḥ   is pronounced with repetition of the preceding vowel e.g. aḥ = aha

ṁ   precedes a consonant

ṅ   precedes k or g.

ṛ   pronounced as ru or ri

c   pronounced as ch

Index

Glossary

Adrenals — endocrine glands producing hormones which control water, mineral and glucose metabolism

Angina Pectoris — pain in the heart region due to coronary artery spasm

Arrhymias — irregular heart beats

Arthritis — inflammation of the joints

Astride — with legs wide apart

Autonomic — pertaining to the sympathetic and parasympathetic nervous system (autonomic nervous system) which are not under voluntary control

Autosuggestion — self suggestion

Bronchiectasis — respiratory disease characterized by chronic dilatation of the bronchial tubes

Calves — back muscles of the lower legs

Cervical — pertaining to the neck

Colitis — inflammation of the colon

Congestion — excessive blood accumulation

Convalescence — recovering from an illness

Diabetes — disease due to deficiency of insulin

Diaphragm — strong muscle separating thoracic and abdominal cavities

Dyspepsia — poor digestion

Emphesema — respiratory disease where the air vesicles in the lungs are dilated

Endocrine gland — ductless glands where the hormone is liberated directly into the blood stream

Eructations — an act of belching

Exhale — to breathe out

Flatulence — excessive gas in the digestive tract

Gallbladder — abdominal organ producing bile

Gastro-intestinal — pertaining to the stomach and intestines

Genitals — external sex organs

Gonads — sex glands: ovaries and testes

Hypertension — high blood pressure

Hyperthyroidism — overfunctioning of the thyroid gland

Hypothalamus — part of the fore brain which regulates the autonomic nervous system

Idiopathic — of unknown origin

Immune — defense

Inhale — to breathe in

Insomnia — inability to sleep

Islets of Langerhans — endocrine glands which produce insulin hormone which controls the blood sugar level

Kumbhaka — retention or stoppage of breath after inhalation or exhalation

Laryngitis — inflammation of the larynx

Larynx — voice box

Lumbodorsal — lumbar and thoracic

Menstrual — pertaining to monthly periods of vaginal bleeding in females

Nadi — very fine channels of the subtle body through which pranic energy flows

Neurosis — mental disorder

Obesity — excess of fat

Oedema — swelling of tissues caused by fluid retention

Ovaries — female sex glands

Pancreas — abdominal organ producing pancreatic enzymes and containing the Islets of Langerhans which produce insulin

Parathyroids — endocrine glands producing hormones controlling calcium and phosphorous metabolism

Paravertebral — next to the vertebral column

Paripurna — full

Pelvic— pertaining to the pelvis

Pelvis — Three bones containing within it a basin shaped cavity situated just below the abdomen

Peptic — pertaining to the stomach and duodenum

Phobias — fears

Pineal — endocrine gland secreting hormones which regulate the acitivity of pituitary and the hypothalamus

Pituitary — master endocrine gland which secretes hormones controlling other endocrine glands

Postural — related to posture

Prāṇāyāma — yogic tecnique of controlling the breath

Prostate — accessory male sex gland situated around the urethra

Pubis — one of the three bones of the pelvis situated in the front of pelvis

Rectum — lower end of the large intestine

Rhinitis — cold in the nose

Sālamba — with support

Slip disc — protrusion of the inter-vertebral cartilaginous disc

Śodhana — purifying

Spinal — related to the spinal cord

Spondylitis — arthritis of vertebral joints

Squat — sit on one's heels

Stammering — speech disorder

Sternum — bone in front of chest where the ribs are attached

Supta — in lying position

Testes — male sex glands

Thoracic — pertaining to the thorax

Thymus — endocrine gland producing hormones concerned in defense of the body

Thyroid — endocrine gland secreting growth controlling hormone

Tonsillitis — inflammation of the tonsils

Tragus — small projection of cartilage covered with skin in front of the ear

Ujjāyī — prolongation

Ūrdhva — raised

Utthita— stretched

Vasomotor — pertaining to the autonomic nervous system

Visceroptosis — sagging of organs

Further Reading

Light on Yoga, B. K. S. Iyengar. Allen and Unwin, 1966.

Light on Prāṇāyāma, B. K. S. Iyengar. Allen and Unwin, 1981.

Yoga A Gem for Women, Geeta S. Iyengar. Allied Publishers Private Ltd. 1983.

The Art of Yoga, B. K. S. Iyengar. Allen and Unwin 1985.

The Tree of Yoga, B. K. S. Iyengar. Shambhala Publications, Inc. 1988.

Light on the Yoga Sutras of Patanjali, B. K. S. Iyengar. The Aquarian Press 1993.